Nutrition in general practice:
giving advice to women

Nutrition in general practice: giving advice to women

Nicola Seabrook BSc, SRD

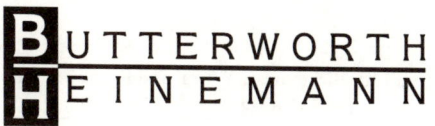

Butterworth-Heinemann
Linacre House, Jordan Hill, Oxford OX2 8DP
A division of Reed Educational and Professional Publishing Ltd

$\mathcal{R}$ A member of the Reed Elsevier plc group

OXFORD   BOSTON   JOHANNESBURG
MELBOURNE   NEW DELHI   SINGAPORE

First published 1997

© Reed Educational and Professional Publishing Ltd 1997

British Library Cataloguing in Publication Data
A catalogue record for this book is available from the British Library

Library of Congress Cataloguing in Publication Data
A catalogue record for this book is available from the Library of Congress

ISBN 0 7506 3464 2

Typeset by Wilmaset Ltd, Birkenhead, Wirral and Printed and bound in Great Britain
by Biddles Ltd, Guildford and Kings Lynn

Contents

To the reader

This book is intended primarily for use by qualified health professionals who have had some training in the field of medicine and nutrition. While most patients can benefit from the advice presented in this book, some patients, such as those with renal disease, may not and thus may require specialist dietary treatment. In all instances readers should use their own clinical discretion as to whether a particular piece of advice is appropriate for the patient in their care. If in any doubt patients should be referred to a dietitian.

Acknowledgements

I should like to thank Mary Cronk, midwifery tutor, for her support with the chapter on Pregnancy; and my brother, Dr Richard Barton, for his help with the chapter on recurrent thrush. My thanks also go to the primary care teams at Ivry Street and Barrack Lane General Practices in Ipswich, whose enthusiasm was a great inspiration to me as I started this book.

Introduction

This book has been written for practice nurses, health visitors, midwives, dietitians and GPs who are regularly involved in giving dietary advice to women. However, any health professional, interested in the role of diet in medicine, may also find this a useful resource.

While drug therapy continues to have an important role in primary medicine, many patients welcome the chance to manage their health personally, using more natural means and, today, nursing staff are frequently called upon to give nutritional advice for a variety of conditions. In the last 10 years there has been a wealth of research published about women's health and nutrition and this has brought some exciting information: we now know how important nutrition is around the time of conception; about the link between growth in the womb and the future health of adults; about the nutrient deficiencies in women with pre-menstrual syndrome and about the importance of calcium in achieving a peak bone mass to name just a few developments. Transforming this information into clinical practice is not always easy and can take time: one of the aims of this book is to try to enhance this process so that many more women can benefit from more up-to-date information.

To help readers, the text has been written in a direct style with few embellishments and for those who are too busy to read the actual text a summary of the key points can be found at the end of each chapter. All the information is based on scientific research and key references are presented alongside the text with full details at the end of each chapter.

Nursing is ultimately about helping people to put medical theory into practice and at the end of each chapter there are one or two case studies to illustrate how this can be done. They are based on personal experiences in general practice, but do not relate exactly to any individuals.

About the chapters

The choice of subjects which have been included in the book are all conditions experienced by large numbers of women in the UK today. They are conditions about which many nurses and GPs receive questions and are also areas in which a substantial amount of research has been carried out. It would, for example, have been of interest to have included a chapter on the menopause but, unfortunately, there is virtually no scientific research on this subject relating to diet, at present.

The first chapter is on obesity and can be referred to for the treatment of both men and women. Obesity is the greatest and perhaps one of the most controversial health problems in our society: the number of people suffering from this condition continues to increase and in this chapter the reader is presented with new ideas about its treatment as well as more established ones. Two diets are available in the appendix at the back and it is intended that anyone working with obese patients can photocopy these and use them in the surgery.

The following chapters are on health issues of specific relevance to women such as pre-menstrual syndrome, recurrent vaginal thrush, coronary heart disease in women, osteoporosis and cancer, including breast cancer. This is then followed by a chapter on irritable bowel syndrome which can be referred to when treating both men and women. This condition is seen frequently in general practice and when dietary advice is given appropriately, it can be very helpful.

The next three chapters: preconception, infertility and pregnancy look at the role of nutrition in reproduction and are particularly relevant to those working in midwifery. The importance of nutrition around the time of conception cannot be stressed enough and the chapter on preconception looks at the work of Wendy Doyle whose research on maternal nutrient intakes and infant birth outcomes highlights this.

Following this there are chapters on how to help low income families choose a healthy diet, the special nutritional needs of ethnic minority groups and finally how patients respond to advice and decide whether or not to change their lifestyle. It should be emphasized that this chapter has not been put at the end because it is any less important than the others and all those using the book are urged to read it. The process of behaviour change in adults is an interesting one and one that everyone should be aware of, if they wish to be effective health educators.

Chapter 1
Treating obesity

Introduction

The subject of obesity is particularly controversial; what appears on the surface to be a straightforward health problem is in fact very complex, and treatment is very difficult. Large numbers of people are suffering from obesity today, more than ever before and it is important that there is a wide network of professional help available for these people to turn to. While dietitians, especially those based within the general practice setting, can help some patients, the large numbers involved strongly supports the case for other health professionals to be trained to help as well.

Nurses working within the community, in well person clinics, diabetic clinics, well woman clinics, family planning clinics and antenatal clinics are ideally placed to help patients with their weight. There is still much misunderstanding about what constitutes a sensible and successful diet, despite a good deal of media attention about body weight, and the medical and nursing professions, whose opinion is greatly valued by patients, must continue to supply patients with accurate information.

This chapter sets out the theory and practice of treating obesity and tries to answer some of the questions which are commonly asked about the best way to lose weight. It also provides two diet plans which can be offered to obese and overweight patients who request a diet sheet. The information in this chapter is, unlike following chapters, intended to be of use to both women and men.

The facts about obesity

Definition of obesity

Obesity is characterized by the excessive store of fatty tissue in the body and is defined as a body mass index (BMI) of more than 30 (BMI $> 30 \text{ kg/m}^2$).

Obesity is clearly linked to poor health, with obese people being more likely to suffer from diabetes, hypertension, cardiovascular disease, certain cancers and osteoarthritis in their weight-bearing joints than people of normal weight (Garrow, 1988). However, for patients who are simply overweight (defined as a BMI between 25–30), as opposed to obese, the risks are much less. Bray (1992) has proposed five categories of BMI and has set out the health risks associated with each of them (Table 1.1).

Table 1.1   Classification of obesity (Garrow, 1981)

Grade	BMI (kg/m^2)	Health risk
0	20–24.9	Very low
I	25–29.9	Low
II	30–39.9	Moderate
III	> 40	Severe
IV	35–39.9	High
V	> 40	Very high

Numbers of patients suffering from obesity

The number of people who are obese in the UK is rising. Unfortunately, health education campaigns over the past two decades have failed to reduce the number of people who are obese and since the beginning of the 1980s the figures have doubled (Table 1.2).

Table 1.2   The increasing prevalence of obesity in the UK adult population (16–64 years)

	1980[1]		1986/87[2]		1993[3]	
	Men	Women	Men	Women	Men	Women
Obese BMI > 30	6%	8%	8%	12%	13%	16%

Reprinted from the British Dietectic Association position paper on the treatment of obesity 1995.
[1]Rosebaum et al., 1985; [2]Gregory et al., 1990; [3]Bennett et al., 1995

Opinion is divided as to why the problem is increasing. Is it because of the changes that have occurred in our diet? Or is it because we are not taking enough exercise? These are the two main areas of discussion and although we do not know the answer yet, the trend towards an increasingly overweight population suggests that something in our lifestyle is not quite right.

Causes of obesity

Genetic

Obesity is widespread within our culture and affects people of every race, gender and class. It is recognized, however, that certain cultures and social classes are more prone to obesity than others and while some social factors can be found to explain this, there are some scientists who feel there is a strong hereditary factor which may account for the predisposition to obesity seen in some groups and individuals.

Certainly, a recognition of this genetic susceptibility can help those working with obese patients to have a greater understanding and sympathy for their condition. However, it does not mean that help is any different and dietary advice should be given with the same enthusiasm to these patients, as to those who have no family history of weight problems.

Diet

Long-term studies show that the majority of people are able to regulate their body weight quite efficiently and that during their life time their weight never varies by more than 10 kg (Garrow, 1981). This fine regulation is brought about by the work of the hypothalamus, a gland situated in the brain which sends out signals to the body telling it when it is hungry and when it is full. This mechanism works very well for the majority of people but is obviously failing in others. There are many reasons put forward for this, but one reason which has much scientific support suggests that it may have something to do with the rich diet we are now consuming.

Over the last 50 years our intake of fat has increased dramatically while our intake of carbohydrate has fallen (MAFF, 1940–1994), and many scientists believe that the mechanisms described above, which regulate energy balance cannot cope when there is this high percentage of fat in the diet (Prentice and Jebb, 1995). The idea that the hypothalamic mechanism breaks down when a rich diet is being consumed was first demonstrated in laboratory rats. When these animals were fed their normal rat chow their pattern of growth was very predictable, however, when they were fed a diet of chocolate, spam and cornflakes their regulatory mechanism failed to work and as a result they overate, becoming obese.

Similar experiments have been carried out upon human beings and generally speaking it has been found that a diet high in fat is less satiating than one which is high in carbohydrates, especially among people with a tendency to obesity (Blundell *et al.*, 1993; Rolls *et al.*, 1994). In other words, it is much easier for people to consume a high calorie intake when they are eating foods which are high in fat and still not feel full. This is easy to understand when we consider how much easier it is to eat foods such as chocolates, crisps and cakes and not feel full, compared with eating a large jacket potato and several portions of vegetables.

The problem with a high fat diet is that not only is it very high in calories but it is also very low in fibre and it is now recognized that fibre is very important in helping the body to regulate its weight. In a famous experiment carried out in Ireland, a group of men were told that they could eat all they wanted to *after* they had consumed 2 kg of potatoes each day; after a 3-month period, most of the men had lost weight and the researchers concluded that when a high intake of unrefined carbohydrate such as this is eaten each day, it leaves little room in the stomach for any high calorie foods and so helps the body to regulate its weight.

Today the average intake of fibre is around 12–13 g per day while in developing countries it is between 40–60 g per day.

Energy intake

Since the 1970s the average energy intake has actually fallen and scientists are now questioning whether the increasing prevalence of obesity is simply related to energy intake or whether it is related to a lack of energy expenditure or the quality of our diet (Prentice and Jebb, 1995).

Part of the reason for the reduction in energy intake is due to the increase in consumption of 'diet foods' in which the sugar content has been replaced by an artificial sweetener, and the fat content has been replaced by a mixture of air, water and chemical additives and this has helped to halve the calorific value of many products. However, despite helping to reduce the energy content of peoples' diets these products do not seem to have had any significant beneficial effect on the incidence of obesity.

Exercise

There is a high correlation between the increase in obesity in this country and the sharp fall in activity which can be charted over the past few decades (Prentice and Jebb, 1995). Inactivity has increased at the work place where machines have taken over a lot of heavy manual work, and in the home where labour-saving devices have reduced the need for physical house work. Today, many leisure pursuits are also passive activities such as watching television, playing on computers or going to the pub and figures kept over the past years show that the number of hours people spend watching television has doubled since the 1960s.

The increase in car ownership has also played a significant part in reducing people's activity levels and most people today choose to use their car rather than to walk or cycle a few miles to work or to the shops. Inactivity is reported to be highest amongst social classes IV and V and it has been suggested that this may be the cause of the higher incidence of obesity in this group. It must be remembered, however, that their diets are also generally poorer, and it is more likely that inactivity *plus* a poor quality of diet is responsible for the increased incidence.

Cultural factors

Affluence has brought a great change in the way we view food. Food is no longer simply a basic necessity for life but is now seen as something to enhance life in a variety of ways. People use food to respond to certain situations: they use it to comfort themselves or others, to reward, to entertain, or to escape. Food is no longer consumed just when we feel hungry.

Another cultural change has been the increased accessibility of food. Many supermarkets are now open 12 hours a day and some for 7 days a week and, of course, there are many venues which are open for much of the evening, selling hot food to take away. Advances in the preservation of food such as freezing and canning has also allowed people to keep much larger stocks of food in their houses and today virtually any food can be stored, cooked and eaten in the home within a few minutes, with very little effort. As a result of food being more available, many people have lost the ability to stick to a regular meal pattern and frequently find themselves snacking continuously.

Drugs

Some drugs when taken over a long period of time can result in unwanted weight gain. This is especially true of some of the hormonal preparations taken by women such as the contraceptive pill and hormone replacement therapy. The long-term use of steroids in the treatment of asthma can also lead to weight problems in some patients.

The disadvantages of being obese

The following conditions are associated with obesity (BMI > 30) in men and women:

- Heart disease
- Diabetes
- Osteoarthritis
- Gall stones
- Raised lipid levels
- High blood pressure
- Glucose intolerance

Additional health problems for women

In women, obesity can have a negative effect on certain endocrine functions. The menstrual cycle for example, can be affected and result in anovulatory cycles and infertility. For the majority of women weight loss will help to restore fertility and a normal menstrual cycle (Schindler, 1994). This should be strongly encouraged in any woman thinking of having a baby as women who are obese during their pregnancy have a significantly higher chance of spontaneous abortion and a higher perinatal mortality rate than women who are a normal weight (Garrow, 1981). Obesity is also associated with increased levels of certain hormones, including an increase in the production of androgens. Severely obese women will often suffer from hirsutism. High circulating levels of oestradiol and insulin found in obese women are thought to be responsible for the high incidence of endometrial cancer in women who are obese (Schindler, 1994). Finally, stress incontinence and other bladder dysfunctions are more common in obese women. Losing weight is important for these women if surgery is to be carried out successfully to correct this.

Social disadvantages

It is the social stigma attached to being overweight that drives most people, particularly young women, to seek advice about losing weight. Society admires and sometimes idolizes those who are slim and as a result many people today are striving by means of exercising or dieting to attain a socially acceptable shape. Most people are very sensitive about their weight and even light-hearted jokes made by colleagues at work or members of the family may be hurtful.

If a patient is severely obese this can become a great handicap to him or her. It may restrict her ability to join in with certain physical activities, dictate which shops she can buy clothes in and also restrict the number of potential partners who are interested in her. Some obese patients may also have problems getting a job. Severe obesity is frequently resented by other members of the family. Children, for instance, may show unhappiness if one of their parents is excessively overweight and may even suggest that they do not attend school functions in order to avoid the embarrassment.

The advantages of losing weight

Apart from the obvious social advantages of losing weight there are many medical ones.

Positive changes to expect with weight loss

- Up to 20% reduction in mortality – particularly for patients with obesity-related health conditions, such as heart disease.
- A reduction in blood pressure.
- A reduction in cholesterol and triglyceride levels.
- Better mobility for those suffering from arthritis.
- A sense of well being.

How to go about helping patients with their weight

While many patients will happily follow a diet on their own, research has shown that patients who receive help from a health professional generally have greater success at losing weight than those who do not (Blackburn, 1993). If a patient attends a clinic then this also allows for her general health to be monitored while she is losing weight; this is advisable in those who have a lot of weight to lose or for those who have health problems such as hypertension, diabetes or any heart disorder. It also allows the nurse to check that she is following the diet correctly and is not taking any short cuts. Abnormal eating patterns often develop if a patient becomes frustrated with a lack of progress and cutting out meals occasionally is very common and needs to be discouraged.

What makes a good reducing diet

Numerous reducing diets are being advertised or recommended by slimming groups and magazines every day and it is useful to know what constitutes a good diet so that you can guide patients when they ask for your
opinion about a new diet.

A good diet is one which:

- Results in a person shedding weight gradually and constantly over a
  long period of time, approximately 0.5–1 kg a week.
- Is nutritionally balanced so that the patient does not become deficient
  in any vitamin or mineral over a period of time.
- Includes regular small quantitites of nutrient rich food (Table 1.3).

Table 1.3   Foods which should be included on a weight-reducing diet

Meat	Cereals
Poultry	Eggs
Vegetables	Dairy products or soya products
Pulses	Fruit
Nuts	

Giving advice to patients following their own weight-reducing diet

Many patients will choose to follow their own weight-reducing diet which
has been recommended to them by a friend or one that they have read about
in a magazine. They may be grateful when attending the practice however,
for your opinion about the diet. The following questions are designed to help
you to do this. If they can answer yes to all the questions below then the
chances are that the diet is a balanced, healthy one.

Check the following:

1 Is the patient having three meals a day?
2 Does the diet include some fibre?
3 Is a variety of foods being eaten?
4 Is it low in fat?
5 Does it include some protein at two out of the three meals?

If a patient says 'no' to any of these questions then you can assume that the
diet is probably not very balanced and should not be followed for a long
period of time.

Two diets to use with patients in the practice

Some patients will specifically ask practice nurses or health visitors for a weight-reducing diet sheet because attempts to lose weight on their own have been unsuccessful. I have included a choice of two diets (see Appendix) which I have found to be successful and which can be tried with patients in the practice. All patients should be tried with the first diet and most will find that they can successfully lose weight while following this. However, there may be patients who do not experience any significant progress with it and they may find the second diet more successful.

The second diet is a diet which is low in gluten. There is increasing evidence that some people are unable to tolerate large amounts of gluten in their diet without suffering from a variety of symptoms, (Levine, Anderson and Levitt, 1981; Catassi *et al.*, 1994; Robbana-Barnat and Fradin 1997) and the first diet, being high in gluten may make some patients feel unwell and be ineffective at helping them lose weight. In particular, any patient who experiences a lot of wind, loose bowel movements or general abdominal distension whilst on the first diet is likely to be a good candidate for the low gluten diet. This diet is virtually free of wheat – the main source of gluten in our diet, with the exception of two slices of white bread allowed at midday for practical reasons. The rest of the diet is made up of carbohydrate from non-gluten containing foods such as corn, potatoes and rice and their associated products such as cornflakes and rice cakes. Patients should have a good intake of fruit and vegetables as well, to ensure that they are having an adequate intake of fibre. (Both diets can be copied from the Appendix at the back of the book.)

Commonly asked questions

Is breakfast important?

Yes, breakfast is important. After the body has gone without food over night a person's metabolic rate is at a very low level and food has the effect of raising it by as much as 20%. If patients are unable to face a full breakfast they should at least have a drink and be encouraged to have a piece of fruit.

Does exercise help weight loss?

Surprisingly most studies have failed to show that exercise accelerates the rate at which weight is lost when patients are also following a diet (Garrow, 1981). This, however, should not deter patients who are moderately overweight from taking some exercise each week. Physical activity has many benefits for the overweight patient: first, it helps to preserve muscle mass which is important for the patient in the long term, secondly, it has a positive effect on blood glucose levels (in the same way that losing weight does) and thirdly it increases a person's level of fitness which can greatly enhance the way a patient feels about themselves.

Exercise increases the amount of energy expended each day, and helps to conserve the amount of muscle tissue present in the body. Muscle tissue helps to give the body strength, tone and definition and has a higher metabolic rate than fatty tissue. Therefore patients should be encouraged to exercise according to their ability, two to three times a week. Swimming, cycling and walking are the most popular forms of exercise in the UK as they do not require a lot of skill and are fairly inexpensive. Some patients may be interested in starting a fitness training programme at a local gym or taking part in a regular sporting activity such as tennis, squash or aerobics.

If patients feel that they have too little time or not enough money to do these activities they should think about increasing their daily exercise by leaving the car at home and walking or cycling to work. This is an excellent way to get regular exercise, save some money, and help the environment all at the same time!

Does exercise increase a person's appetite or suppress it?

There is no significant research to suggest that moderate exercise has either effect on human beings (Garrow, 1981). During the time when a person is actively exercising and for a short time afterwards their desire for food is often suppressed but feelings of hunger usually return shortly afterwards and food intake over a 24-hour period regains its normal pattern.

Does repeated dieting result in a lower metabolic rate?

Many health professionals are concerned that men and women who spend much of their lives dieting are at risk of experiencing a progressive fall in metabolic rate. At present, however, there is no scientific evidence to support this concern and short-term studies of weight cycling – where women spend alternate weeks dieting and then eating normally – show that metabolic rates do not fall (Jebb et al., 1991).

Why do women gain weight before their period?

Some women gain 1.4–2 kg before they menstruate and this is due to an increase in the amount of water that is being retained by the body. For most women the fluid is evenly distributed and does not bother them. For some women, however, the gain is very uncomfortable and is accompanied by symptoms of breast tenderness and abdominal bloating. Avoiding caffeinated drinks and salt in the diet can help some women to reduce the amount of fluid they retain each month (Abraham, 1984).

Does the contraceptive pill cause women to gain weight?

Weight gain is a common side effect of the oral contraceptive pill, although few studies have been carried out to show this or investigate why this happens. Some women notice an immediate weight gain when they start the pill and if this is the case a lower dose pill is usually recommended, particularly if they are having other side effects as well. For others the weight gain can happen gradually over a number of years and women may not attribute it to the pill. Why or how this happens is not really known. One commonly held belief is that women on the pill experience an increase in appetite. In a recent study carried out to look at appetite and the pill, researchers reported that women had noticeably lower levels of the satiety hormone cholecystokinin when they were given the pill compared to the levels measured before the pill was taken. Cholecystokinin is a hormone which suppresses the desire for food and if levels were low in the body this would naturally lead women to feel more hungry. This is only one theory, however, and more research is needed in this area before any conclusions can be drawn.

Reasons why patients fail to lose weight

It is relatively easy for patients to lose weight while they are an inpatient on a metabolic ward. This has been proved by many people, including Professor Garrow, an expert in the field of obesity, who has recorded the successful weight loss of many patients admitted to a metabolic ward where they were given 1705 ml (3 pints) milk a day plus a daily vitamin and iron supplement. This, however, is an artificial setting and an artificial dietary regimen and does not help us understand why people fail to lose weight when they are at home. The pressures at home and at work to eat foods which are not part of a prescribed diet are considerable. Here are a few of them:

- Food is very accessible today and is quickly prepared in many instances.
- The advertising of food on television encourages people to eat between meals.
- Many of our social activities are associated with eating and it is very difficult for overweight people to refuse food on these occasions.
- Work colleagues may actually encourage people to break their diet through jealousy or resentment that their colleague may be developing a better figure than them.
- There is always pressure at weekends and on holidays to abandon a diet.
- Certain life pressures make it difficult for people to keep to a routine.

Women and family dynamics

Trying to keep to a diet while shopping and cooking for a family who demand and can cope with a more indulgent, normal diet can bring additional pressures for women. They become providers of food that they themselves have to refuse on a daily basis and for some women this regular act of self-denial is impossible. The alternative is for the whole family to be denied luxury foods, but this is not a sacrifice that most women would wish to put their families through.

Most women who look after a family are commonly reported to put their children and husbands first and themselves last and this behaviour can also hinder their success. For example, many women will not put aside low calorie food such as fruit and yoghurts for themselves, but let their children eat them first and end up breaking their diet with a biscuit or piece of cake when they are hungry. This could be because many women are anxious that their diet should intrude as little as possible upon their family. Following a diet has overtones of being preoccupied with oneself rather than the family and to avoid this image, many women will go out of their way to ensure that their family are not affected at all.

At a deeper level, there may be clear psychological reasons why women fail to lose weight and this is discussed in some depth in Susie Orbach's first book called, *Fat is a Feminist Issue* (1986). In her book she describes how some women fail to lose weight because they see their weight as a form of protection against the sexual advances of men, or for others their additional weight has become a positive thing, giving them a feeling of physical strength and power.

Therefore, if women have been unsuccessful at losing weight for many years or seem reticent to follow a diet, it may be because they have some underlying psychological factor which needs to be addressed. In this case some sensitive questioning and offer of help from a psychiatric nurse may be much more valuable than dietary advice.

Slimming products

Artificial sweeteners

Artificial sweeteners are used by many people trying to lose weight. They are commonly added to hot drinks and breakfast cereals and allow people to satisfy their sweet tooth. Some people buy manufactured products which contain artificial sweeteners as well, for example, sugar-free fruit yoghurts, jellies, mousses, squashes and fizzy drinks.

By substituting a sweetener for the sugar in a product, the number of calories can be reduced quite significantly and this is a great attraction to many people. Unfortunately, however, there is no evidence from long-term studies to suggest that people who use artificially sweetened foods are able to control their weight any more successfully than people who use sugar and some research suggests that they may actually encourage people to eat more.

One study has shown that both naturally sweet and artificially sweet foods will stimulate a person's appetite (Rogers and Blundell, 1989). The study also showed that because artificially sweetened foods are so low in energy and poor at satisfying hunger, a person is more likely to increase her food intake over the next few hours to make up for it. As a result people will consume the same number of calories or more, as occurred in the experiment, than they would have done if they had eaten a plain starchy meal at the beginning.

Conclusion
Artificial sweeteners may be useful in the short term to help people cut down on their sugar intake but in the long term they should be discouraged and replaced with more naturally sweetened products. Sugar-free desserts do not have to be sweetened with an artificial sweetener but can be sweetened with fruit. For example, natural yoghurt with stewed fruit or plain fromage frais with fresh fruit makes a healthier dessert than an artificially sweetened yoghurt. In the winter baked apples sweetened with dried fruit and a toasted oat cereal served with a little single cream is very good. These desserts will provide a person with some sustaining energy and should not mean that they are searching in the food cupboards half an hour later.

Low fat products

Low fat products such as low fat milks, low fat spreads and low fat cheeses are useful alternative dairy products for anyone trying to lose weight. Fat is a highly calorific nutrient which contains 9 kcal/g (carbohydrate contains 4 kcal/g and protein 4 kcal/g). Therefore anyone trying to reduce their energy intake should begin by restricting the amount of fat they have in their diet.

The overall fat content of a person's diet must be taken into account, however, and if a patient does not like skimmed or semi-skimmed milk it may be more productive to get them to think about choosing grilled meat rather than meat pies or a chicken kebab rather than a donner kebab on a Saturday night!

Meal replacements

Many women who are unsuccessful at losing weight on conventional diets try meal replacements. These are usually milk-based drinks or biscuits which are supplemented with vitamins and minerals and are meant to be as nutritionally complete as a cooked meal. They usually contain between 100 and 225 kcal and are designed to replace two out of the three meals each day. Patients are meant to have one cooked meal a day while they are taking these. Unfortunately these products are not as healthy as they appear. In a report published by the Food Commission, most meal replacements were found to be high in sugar and fat and low in protein and *not* significantly lower in calories when compared with ordinary cereal bars or sweetened milk drinks (Dibb, 1992).

Meal replacements do not help to re-educate a patient's eating habits and it is now thought that the twice daily intake of a highly sweetened drink or biscuit may actually perpetuate a person's desire for sugary foods. An additional concern about meal replacements is that many advertise that women can lose between 2–3 kg a week while using them. This is not recommended by experts in the medical profession who recommend a weekly loss of between 0.5–1 kg.

In summary therefore, meal replacements are not recommended unless all else has failed and the patient's health is almost certainly likely to benefit from the weight loss, i.e. they have a body mass of more than 30.

The role of the dietitian

Dietitians have a lot of experience to offer overweight patients and anyone who does not respond to conventional dietary advice should be referred to a dietitian. They have time to assess the relevant medical risk factors, discuss a patient's dieting history, assess a person's energy requirements and perhaps most importantly assess a patient's ability and readiness to make lifestyle changes. They may also be able to offer specialist dietary advice. Most dietitians see patients on a one-to-one basis, but some dietitians who have a special interest in obesity may be willing to help set up and lead a slimming group within the practice.

Setting up a slimming clinic

Some patients feel that attending a slimming group is the best way for them to lose weight but commercial clubs can be expensive. Many men and women enjoy exchanging ideas about their diet in a group setting and can feel more motivated when they have to be weighed each week in front of their peer group. As well as giving motivation, a group can often provide support as well. Therefore, if there is a spare room at the surgery in the evenings and two members of staff are keen, a slimming group can be set up to help overweight patients in the practice. Dietitians are usually happy to come and lead the first few sessions and in many cases offer long-term support to the group.

To encourage patients to attend regularly it is important to make meetings as imaginative as possible. Here are some ideas for weekly sessions:

● Health education videos: these can be hired together with a video player from the Health Education Authority.
● Visiting speakers, e.g. psychologist, keep fit instructor.
● Cookery demonstrations (if facilities are available).
● Discussions about other relevant health topics, e.g. how to feed a family healthy food on a budget, eating to prevent osteoporosis, and diet and heart disease.

The success of group therapy compared to individual counselling has been reviewed and the results have been mixed with some studies showing them to be more successful than individual counselling and others less. Certainly anyone who is considering setting up a group needs to be committed and enthusiastic for it to work and they need to have some support from another nurse or health professional.

The advantages of group therapy include:

● It is economical with your time – many patients can be seen all together at the same time.
● Patients should receive more information if they attend most of the

sessions compared with someone attending a few short individual consultations.

- Mutual support from other members within the group can be very valuable. Mutual support from group members is only likely to come about if patients from a similar background or with similar interests attend. Organizing this may be rather difficult to achieve but should be considered as it is important if the group is to gel. (Single sex groups may be more successful in this respect.)
- An evening session is often preferred by those who work rather than having to keep day time appointments.
- Alternative methods of communication can be used which are more accessible to patients, e.g. videos, food tasting, speakers, patient led discussions, etc.

Choosing your group of patients for a slimming group

Apart from choosing patients from a similar social background or with a similar lifestyle (e.g. young mothers with pre-school children or retired men), another way of increasing the success of a group is to select patients with characteristics that are more likely to succeed. A review of the literature on the subject suggests that patients who are most successful at losing weight share similar characteristics (Pearson, de Looy and Webster, 1989).

These are patients who are:

- Over 40 years old.
- With a medical condition that will improve with weight loss.
- With a BMI less than 35.

Age is an important factor: people over 40 are usually more motivated by health issues than younger patients and as a result are more willing to change their eating patterns. This does not mean that young people should be excluded from health education programmes, but simply that those who are involved in running them recognize that programmes for young people may be less successful.

Anyone who is overweight and has a medical condition such as hypertension, diabetes or osteoarthritis will benefit from losing some weight and for many people over 40 this is what motivates them to try a reducing diet. It is not known why those with a BMI over 35 do not tend to do as well. Patients with a BMI over 35 are classed as having severe obesity and the causes of it may be more complex.

Helping patients to maintain their weight loss

Helping patients to maintain their weight once they have achieved a desirable target is not an easy task. Most studies show that there is a tendency for people to gain weight after a period of dieting and for their weight to return to the original measurement (Garner and Wooley, 1991).

However, a study in Finland which looked at the outcome of a weight-reduction course, led by some nurses based at health centres, found that the long-term results were not too disappointing especially in men. Seven years after the initial advice 53% of the men still weighed 10 kg less than their original weight, while for women the figure was 21%. This level of weight reduction would certainly be sufficient to improve the mortality and morbidity of all patients with mild to moderate obesity. These results were in contrast to the control group who received no weight-reduction advice and who gained weight during the first year (Table 1.4).

In conclusion therefore it does appear that a significant weight loss can be achieved and maintained by a substantial number of people.

Table 1.4   Average weight loss (kg) in patients after attending a 6-week weight-reduction programme in a Finnish primary care setting

Numbers	Male (22)	Female (71)	Male (control) (20)	Female (control) (76)
After 1 year	10.9	5.4	+0.9	+0.2
After 7 years	8.7	3.5	Not measured	Not measured

Karvetti and Hakala (1992)

Summary

Obesity is the largest nutritional problem in the UK at present. The reasons for this are many but it does appear that the high fat, low fibre diet that many people are eating is a contributing factor, along with low levels of exercise.

Nurses and dietitians could share this work effectively, providing patients with a choice of individual or group counselling within the surgery. Dietary advice should always aim to help patients achieve a balanced food intake and for the majority this will entail following a low sugar, low fat, high fibre diet. There is a need however to be flexible and where patients are experiencing discomfort in the form of various bowel symptoms they should be tried on a low wheat fibre diet.

Key points – dietary advice

- Ask patients to reduce their fat intake
- Make sure that all foods containing sugar have been cut out
- Check that a patient has an adequate intake of fibre from cereals, bread, fruit and vegetables
- Check a patient's alcohol intake
- If the patient is doing all the above but is not having any success they may find that a low wheat fibre diet suits them better.

References

Abraham, G. E. (1984) Nutrition and the premenstrual syndromes. *Journal of Applied Nutrition*, **36**, 103–124

Bennet, N., Dodd, T., Flatley, J. *et al.* (1995) *Health Survey for England 1993*. London: HMSO

Blackburn, G. L. (1993) Comparison of medically supervised and unsupervised approaches to weight loss and control (review paper). *Annals of Internal Medicine*, **7**, 714–718

Blundell, J. E., Burley, V. J., Cotton, J. R. *et al.* (1993) Dietary fat and control of energy intake: evaluating the effect of fat on meal size and post-meal satiety. *American Journal of Clinical Nutrition*, **57**, 772–785

Catissi, C., Ratschi-M., Fabiani, E. *et al.* (1994) Coeliac disease in the year 2000: exploring the iceberg. *Lancet*, **343**, 200

Dibb, S. (1992) The slimming scandal. *The Food Magazine*, **2**, 8–9.

Garner, D. M. and Wooley, S. C. (1991) Confronting the failure of behavioural and dietary treatments of obesity. *Clinical Psychology Review*, **6**, 58–137

Garrow, J. (1981) *Treat Obesity Seriously: a Clinical Manual*. Edinburgh: Churchill Livingstone

Garrow, J. (1988) *Obesity and Related Diseases*. Edinburgh: Churchill Livingstone

Gregory, J., Foster, K., Tyler, H. *et al.* (1990) *The Dietary and Nutritional Survey of British Adults*. London: HMSO

Jebb, S. A., Goldberg, G. R., Coward, W. A. *et al.* (1991) Effects of weight cycling caused by intermittent dieting on metabolic rate and body composition in obese women. *International Journal of Obesity*, **15**, 74

Karvetti, R. L. and Hakala, P. (1992) A seven year follow-up of a weight reduction programme in Finnish primary health care. *European Journal of Clinical Nutrition*, **46**, 743–752

Levine, A., Anderson, I. H. and Levitt, M. (1981) Incomplete absorption of the carbo-hydrate in all-purpose wheat flour. *New England Journal of Medicine*, **304** (15), 891–892

Ministry of Agriculture Fisheries and Foods (1940–1994) *Household Food Consumption and Expenditure*. London: HMSO

Orbach, S. (1986) *Fat is a Feminist Issue*. London: Arrow Books

Pearson, G. C., de Looy, A. E. and Webster, J. (1989) Analysis of the dietetic treatment of obesity. *Journal of Human Nutrition and Dietetics*, **2**, 371–378

Prentice, A. and Jebb, S. (1995) Obesity in Britain: gluttony or sloth? *British Medical Journal*, **311**, 437–439

Robbana-Barnat, S. and Fradin, J. (1997) Cereal grains: IgE- and Non-IgE-medicated reactions. *Journal of Nutritional and Environmental Medicine*, **7**(1), 35–46

Rogers, P. J. and Blundell, J. E. (1989) Separating the actions of sweetness and calories: effects of saccharin and carbohydrates on hunger and food intake in human subjects. *Physiology and Behaviour*, **45**, 1093–1099

Rolls, B. J., Lim-Haio, S., Fischman, M. W. *et al.* (1994) Satiety after pre-loads with different amounts of fat and carbohydrate: implications for obesity. *American Journal of Clinical Nutrition*, **60**, 476–487

Rosenbaum, S., Skinner, R. J., Knight, I. B. *et al.* (1985) A survey of heights and weights of adults in Great Britain. *Annals of Human Biology*, **12**, 115–127

Schindler, A. E. (1994) Obesity: health hazard for women. *Current Obstetrics and Gynaecology*, **4**, 37–40

Wooley, S. and Garner, D. (1994) Dietary treatments for obesity are ineffective. *British Medical Journal*, **309**, 654–656

Further reading

Dibb, S. (1991) Can diet products help you slim? *The Food Magazine*, **2**, 20

Garrow, J. S. (1994) Should obesity be treated? *British Medical Journal*, **309**, 654–656

The Food Magazine (1992) The Slimming Scandal. **2**, 1, 8–9

Chapter 2

Pre-menstrual syndrome

Introduction

Pre-menstrual syndrome is believed to affect between 20 and 50% of women in the UK and approximately half of all gynaecological referrals are concerned with this condition. The degree to which women are affected by the symptoms of pre-menstrual syndrome (PMS) varies greatly, with some women experiencing unbearable symptoms each month and others simply being aware that they feel slightly off colour.

The exact cause and pathophysiology of PMS is still unknown and the only statement which has any consensus among scientists and the medical profession is that PMS is a function of cyclical ovarian activity (Magos, 1990). Beyond this basic preface however, there is a great deal of disagreement and uncertainty.

The lack of a clinical definitive answer about the cause of PMS has unfortunately left the medical profession unsure how to treat it and very often resorting to the prescription of treatments which do not have substantial, unequivocal scientific evidence to support their use. For example, there is a large amount of data which show that some of the traditional therapies such as progesterone, progestogens, pyridoxine, bromocryptine, and diuretics are ineffective (Magos, 1990) and, as a result, patients are often disappointed by the results.

In the last decade progesterone has been widely used to treat PMS and Dr Dalton, a pioneer of treatment for PMS, has written about the success she has had with it (Dalton, 1991). However, several scientific trials, conducted recently, have failed to show that it has any more effect than a placebo, even at high doses (Freeman *et al.*, 1990).

At present the only drugs which are acknowledged to be superior to a placebo are drugs which suppress ovulation including danazol, GnRH analogues and anovulatory doses of oestradiol administered through a subcutaneous implant. However, these drugs can have side effects and not all women benefit from taking them. In a recent surveys of 100 PMS sufferers, 10 said they had been given danazol but only two reported that they had felt better while taking it (Leather *et al.*, 1993).

The limitations of drug therapy are increasingly being recognized by many women and over half of the women in the above survey said that they were prepared to undergo a total hysterectomy to alleviate their symptoms. This is strong evidence of a widespread dissatisfaction with current orthodox therapy.

Nutritional therapy

Against this background of disenchantment with a drug-orientated approach, several practioners, most notably Dr Alan Stewart and Maryon Stewart at the Women's Nutritional Advisory Service (WNAS), have had considerable success treating PMS using dietary therapy and nutritional supplementation. This approach is based on a great deal of research which has been carried out both here and in the USA and which is now gaining support from many medical practitioners and dieticians working in the field of women's health. The primary care team is ideally placed to help women with PMS and this chapter discusses how practice nurses, health visitors and nursing practitioners can identify the symptoms and help women to make the appropriate changes to their diet. Included in the chapter are practical sections on how to give dietary advice to mild sufferers and also how to recognize when a woman, with moderate to severe PMS, may be suffering from a food intolerance. These patients then need to be referred to a dietitian. The use of vitamin and mineral supplements is discussed at the end.

When does PMS occur?

Before looking at how PMS can be treated, it is useful to outline the symptoms of this condition and to discuss how it can affect a woman's life. This can be helpful for those nurses using this book who are fortunate enough not to have experienced PMS, even in its mildest form.

Pre-menstrual syndrome is a collection of symptoms – mental and physical – which can occur up to 14 days before menstruation and which may not clear until the end of menstruation. Most sufferers usually feel ill for 7–10 days before their period and then experience significant relief when menstruation starts. However, a few women do not feel better until the end of their period which means that they can feel ill for 3 out of 4 weeks of every month. PMS can only occur in the reproductive years of a woman's life but it should be noted that symptoms can continue even after a woman has had a hysterectomy, if she has not yet entered the menopause. Pregnancy can bring considerable relief to many women as the symptoms of PMS usually disappear during the second half of pregnancy. Unfortunately they can return with greater severity after the birth and can sometimes be misinterpreted as post-natal depression. PMS will often occur when a woman who has been on the pill for a long time comes off it or after she has experienced a period of amenorrhoea. While it is more common in women over 30, some young girls in their teens can also suffer with it.

Pre-menstrual symptoms

The symptoms that are most commonly associated with PMS are irritability, anxiety, aggression and emotional instability and these are usually the symptoms which women find hardest to bear. There are many other symptoms however that are also part of the syndrome. In the next section the symptoms are divided up into three groups: physical, mental and miscellaneous. Most women experience some physical and mental symptoms each month.

Mental symptoms

- Nervous tension
- Forgetfulness
- Anxiety
- Depression
- Insomnia
- Agoraphobia
- Crying

Physical symptoms

- Abdominal bloating
- Loose bowel movements
- Weight gain
- Mouth ulcers
- Generalized muscle aches
- Mastalgia
- Fatigue
- Acne
- Migraine
- Swelling of extremities

Miscellaneous symptoms

- Sensitivity to noise and light
- Poor libido
- Sugar cravings

The above symptoms are sometimes grouped under four headings – a classification system which was first devised by Dr Guy Abraham, a Professor of Gynaecology in the USA (Abraham and Rumley, 1987). Each of the four subgroups is a group of symptoms which is concerned with a particular aspect of PMS, e.g. sugar cravings or fluid retention or anxiety symptoms. Below are the following subgroups that many books refer to:

PMT – A
This is the commonest subgroup and patients in this group complain chiefly of anxiety, irritability symptoms and nervous tension. Elevated blood oestrogen levels and low progesterone levels have been observed in this group.

PMT – H
Patients in this group complain of excessive weight gain, abdominal bloating, an increased breast size each month, mastalgia and general oedema all over their body. Except in exceptional cases pre-menstrual weight gain is usually less than 1.3 kg.

PMT – C
Patients with PMT – C usually complain of an increased appetite and a craving for sweet things premenstrually. If they give in to these cravings and consume large amounts of cakes, biscuits and chocolate they often feel faint afterwards and experience palpitations, dizziness and headaches.

PMT – D
Patients with PMT – D suffer with depression, feelings of confusion, uncontrollable crying and suicidal feelings. They usually require psychiatric support and fortunately this PMT group is not very common.

Please note: although these subgroups can be helpful in working out the best treatment for a patient, many women experience symptoms in more than one of the subgroups and can rarely be described as just having PMT – A or PMT – H for instance. For this reason I feel that they are of limited value, although it is useful to be aware of them.

The social consequences of PMS

Dr Katarina Dalton has written extensively about pre-menstrual syndrome and how it can affect family life. She has documented the detrimental effect

Table 2.1   Affect of PMS on the lifestyle of 100 women with PMS

	Not applicable	Number affected	Severely affected
Work performance	14	80	27.5
Work relationships	23	70	22.1
Household chores	1	97	45.5
Relationship with partner	6	93	82.8
Relationship with children	22	77	61
Social relationships	2	94	41.5

Reproduced from Leather *et al.* 1993, *Journal of the Royal Society of Medicine* by permission of the Editor

that it can have on a woman's performance at work and how in severe cases it can lead to criminal behaviour. Perhaps most alarming of all is the fact that a woman with untreated PMS can become a danger to her children. In a study of 132 women attending a PMS clinic in 1977, at University College Hospital, London, 6% had been referred because of battering their children (Dalton, 1991).

It is very hard for women to understand why they are experiencing these unnatural feelings each month and many are placed under considerable personal stress because of it. This is borne out by some figures from the latter study in which the author found that 37% of the women who were referred had had a previous mental hospital admission and 34% had attempted suicide or homicide at some time.

In a more recent study, the effects of PMS on family relationships and daily life for 100 women who were referred to a specialist PMS clinic, were documented (Table 2.1). This survey shows how invasive PMS can be – affecting all the major every day activities of women. Even more significantly, it shows the degree to which marital relationships can be affected. Living with a PMS sufferer can be extremely difficult and it is difficult for men to know how to react to women who suddenly become irrational, unreasonable and even aggressive. If this behaviour is occurring for several days of each month, every month, then the relationship may not survive.

Children are also affected by this syndrome, as is shown by the survey and some paediatricians believe that children can become psychologically scarred if they are subjected to years of unprovoked verbal abuse from their mother each month.

In conclusion, the treatment of PMS is essential, not only to restore mental stability and physical well being for women but also so that the normal life of their family has a chance of surviving too.

A nutritional approach to treating PMS

Introduction

In the 1940s Dr Biskind was the first doctor to try treating PMS with a nutritional approach. He suggested that many of the mental symptoms of premenstrual syndrome were similar to those seen when a person has a vitamin B deficiency and he went on to prove that the mental symptoms of pre-menstrual tension could be improved by taking a vitamin B complex supplement every day. Since then a great deal of research and clinical work has been carried out to look at the role of nutrition in treating PMS and there is now a significant amount of scientific evidence to suggest that modifying someone's diet and recommending certain nutrients in a supplementary form can greatly improve and in many cases cure PMS (Abraham and Rumley, 1987; Stewart, 1987; Facchinetti et al., 1991; Stewart, Tooley and Stewart, 1991). In particular, the research has highlighted three points:

1 That women with PMS often have vitamin and mineral deficiencies.
2 That the use of vitamin and mineral supplements can help to improve many PMS symptoms.
3 That certain dietary habits can aggravate the symptoms of PMS.

Vitamin and mineral deficiencies

Multiple nutrient deficiencies were documented by Dr Alan Stewart in 11 women suffering with PMS including low levels of magnesium in red cells and sweat, vitamin B deficiencies and low serum levels of vitamin E and zinc. Other studies have found that women with PMS are frequently deficient in magnesium.

Treatment of PMS with vitamin and mineral supplements

The most extensive research in this area has been carried out using a multivitamin and mineral supplement called Optivite which, with its high concentration of vitamin B_6 and magnesium was specifically designed to treat PMS sufferers. Four open and three double blind trials have found that most women with moderate to severe PMS show significant improvements in their symptoms when 6 Optivite tablets are taken daily over a 3-month period (Abraham and Rumley, 1987). However, this is a very high intake of vitamins and minerals to take and some women can react adversely to the high levels of vitamin B_6 in this preparation and develop peripheral neuropathy. It is therefore not advisable to recommend that women take more than one tablet a day, unless their doctor is aware and in agreement with this. The use of individual vitamins and minerals for PMS will be discussed later in this chapter.

A healthy diet can improve PMS symptoms

As well as taking vitamin supplements most nutrition programmes have found that changing to a healthier diet can be very beneficial and should be part of the treatment as well (Abraham and Rumeley, 1987; Stewart, Tooley and Stewart, 1991). This involves women reducing their intake of caffeine and sugar and increasing their intake of green vegetables, salads, fruit and good quality vegetable oils.

Treating PMS through diet in general practice

Thanks to the clinical experience and enthusiasm of a small group of medical practitioners with a special interest in nutrition, there is now a growing acknowledgement and acceptance by more orthodox practitioners, that diet can play a significant part in the treatment of PMS. Information is gradually filtering down to GPs, dieticians and health visitors working in primary care and some are now very involved in treating women with PMS in this way.

All nurses who work in the community should be able to recognize the symptoms of PMS and feel confident about giving out basic dietary advice to women with mild or moderate symptoms. However, women with severe symptoms should be referred to a dietician, or a medical practitioner who specializes in nutritional medicine, as these patients usually require specialized dietary advice involving the exclusion of certain foods and the correction of significant vitamin and mineral deficiencies.

Practical dietary advice for mild sufferers

Dietary treatment for mild sufferers is simple and straightforward and can be given by health visitors, practice nurses or midwives. The diet can best be described as a sugar-free, high fibre diet and the following section explains how this can be achieved in detail.

All sources of sugar should be avoided in the diet
Patients should be advised to cut out the main sources of sugar in their diet which includes sugar added to drinks or cereals and foods which contain significant amounts of sugar such as cakes, biscuits, chocolate, sweets, desserts and sugar coated cereals. Small amounts of sugar found in cereals such as cornflakes and Weetabix and in savoury foods such as pickles do not need to be avoided.

There should be a good intake of fibre
A good intake of fibre is important for PMS suffers for three reasons: firstly, it enhances the excretion of oestrogen from the body and oestrogen levels can be undesirably high in some PMS sufferers. Secondly, it helps to keep blood sugar levels stable and thirdly, it increases the magnesium content of the diet as foods which are high in fibre are usually high in magnesium and B vitamins as well – both of which are important in the treatment of PMS.

Patients should be encouraged to increase their fibre intake by having three portions of fruit, and two portions of fresh or frozen vegetables each day. They should eat nuts as a snack food in between meals and beans, peas or lentils as a vegetable or main protein source once or twice a week. Whole grain cereals should be encouraged at breakfast and wholemeal bread or a soft grain bread should be used for sandwiches and toast.

An adequate intake of protein should be eaten each day
An adequate intake of protein in the diet is important for women with PMS. Foods which are high in protein, such as meat, cheese, eggs and pulses are very good sources of iron and zinc and these nutrients are often lacking in the diets of women with PMS. Women should be encouraged to have some protein at lunch and in the evening. For example, a white roll and a cup of soup is not really an adequate lunch; this should be replaced by a cheese and salad or ham roll and a piece of fresh fruit.

Women should have small regular meals
Many women with PMS suffer with low blood sugar levels during their premenstrual phase, and this sometimes leads to excessive sweating, palpitations, dizziness and fatigue. These symptoms of hypoglycaemia can be avoided if women have regular healthy meals or snacks. This should also help to curb their strong cravings for something sweet. Small amounts of food should be eaten every 4 hours if possible, even if it is only some fruit or a packet of nuts. Eating a biscuit or some chocolate may boost a person's sugar level in the

short term, but it will not help them to maintain a good blood glucose level in the long term. This should therefore be discouraged.

Caffeine intake should be restricted
Caffeine is a well known stimulant which can aggravate many of the anxiety symptoms of PMS; it can also cause pre-menstrual headaches, breast tenderness and insomnia. Coffee and tea are the main sources of caffeine in our diet with filter and percolated coffee being particularly concentrated sources of caffeine. Patients should be advised to change to decaffeinated coffee and limit their tea intake to two to three cups a day. There are many alternatives to tea and coffee that patients can try, including barley cup, Ovaltine, Bournvita, cocoa and a variety of herbal teas. Encourage your patients to be adventurous!

It should be remembered that anyone who is used to consuming a lot of coffee each day may experience some withdrawal symptoms when they stop, for example, severe headaches and aching limbs. They should be warned of this and given the opportunity of reducing their intake of coffee gradually rather than all at once.

Seeing the patient again
It is important to arrange to see patients after they have followed the diet for 4–6 weeks so that they can ask questions and their progress can be monitored. If their symptoms are less noticeable after the first month they should be encouraged to continue for another month. Patients should notice that as well as becoming less severe their symptoms should last for a shorter time each month. At the end of 3 months they should be almost free from all their symptoms. If patients do not improve it is very likely that an alternative diet will be more suited to their symptoms and the following section gives information on how to help these women.

Helping moderate to severe sufferers

Severe sufferers of PMS or those who do not improve on the advice above, should be screened to see if they have a set of specific symptoms. These symptoms, which are listed below, usually indicate that the patient is suffering from a food intolerance. Nurses can assess which patients with PMS have these symptoms and then refer them to a dietitian for dietetic advice and help with the food intolerance.

In order to decide whether a patient has a food intolerance or not, some time must be spent carefully checking the patient's symptoms. Below is a list of symptoms which are associated with a food intolerance in PMS. The first set is generally associated with a wheat intolerance and the second set associated with a yeast intolerance although this is not always the case.

Symptoms of a wheat intolerance

- Severe mood swings
- Peripheral oedema in the fingers, ankles and face
- Excessive wind
- Mouth ulcers

Symptoms of a yeast intolerance

- Severe mood swings
- Frequent bouts of recurrent thrush
- Headaches
- An intolerance to wine
- Itchy skin.

The patient should be asked if she is suffering from any of these symptoms and if so, it is highly likely that she is suffering from a food intolerance. A dietitian attached to the practice or based at the hospital will be able to help her sort out an appropriate diet and after 3–4 weeks she should be feeling a lot better.

The use of vitamins and minerals to treat PMS

Introduction

Vitamins and minerals can be helpful in the treatment of PMS and given the right supplement and the right dietary advice, most women can feel a lot better and will sustain this improvement for a very long time, if not for ever. It should be stressed, however, that the use of vitamin supplements on their own, without dietary advice is not usually very successful in the long term. Below, is some information on each nutrient which can help to allevi-ate the symptoms of PMS. Each part includes information on when to re-commend the nutrient, what dose should be taken and the dangers of taking too high a dose.

Magnesium

Several research studies have reported that women with PMS have reduced levels of magnesium in their red blood cells when compared with the general population and in one study 45% of patients with PMS had an erythrocyte magnesium level below the normal range (Sherwood *et al.*, 1986). Professor Abraham, an authority on PMS, has suggested that many of the symptoms of PMS may be related to a magnesium deficiency and several trials conducted both by himself and others have demonstrated that a supplement high in magnesium and vitamin B_6 can give good results.

Magnesium is being tried by a number of women today to help their PMS and in a recent study more than one-third of women who had tried it reported that it had been helpful (Leather *et al.*, 1993). If you are considering recommending this mineral to a patient it is useful first to find out if the patient is exhibiting any of the physical symptoms of a magnesium deficiency. If she is, and there is no other medical reason for these symptoms, she is likely to benefit from taking a supplement.

Common physical symptoms of a magnesium deficiency
- Constipation
- Numbness or pins and needles in the limbs
- Uncontrollable flickering of the eyes
- Insomnia
- Weakness and tiredness (Davies and Stewart, 1987).

Dose: magnesium is not a toxic mineral and can be taken in moderate amounts quite safely. Doctors specializing in nutritional medicine recommend patients with PMS take 200–400 mg of magnesium a day. Various forms of magnesium either with or without calcium can be purchased from a health food shop.

Side effects: high doses of magnesium may cause diarrhoea but patients would normally have to take more than 500 mg before this would happen.

Vitamin B_6 (pyridoxine)

Vitamin B_6 has been one of the most popular nutritional treatments for PMS since the beginning of the 1970s and is still prescribed by many GPs today. Some women find their symptoms are relieved when they take this vitamin but many do not and I am of the opinion that without dietary advice as well, vitamin B_6 on its own only has a limited effect.

Dose: as a treatment for PMS, women should be advised to take 50 mg of vitamin B_6 a day for 2–3 months.

Side effects: vitamin B_6 can cause peripheral neuropathy at very high doses and there have been reports of peripheral neuropathy developing among women even when they were taking only 50 mg a day. It seems advisable therefore for women to check with their GP before taking this level of vitamin B_6 each day.

Evening primrose oil

Evening primrose oil contains high concentrations of an essential fatty acid called linoleic acid. This fatty acid along with another one called linolenic acid is involved in many important functions in the body including the production of hormones, the health and vitality of the skin and the inhibition of inflammatory reactions. Patients with PMS who have mastalgia are the group of women most likely to benefit from taking essential fatty acids and preparations of evening primrose oil such as Efamol are now licensed and available on prescription for this condition.

Dose: most women need to take 2000 mg a day to achieve any improvement in their symptoms. Capsules are available in three different strengths: 250 mg, 500 mg and 1000 mg.

Alternatively, women can take star oil which contains about twice the concentration of essential fatty acids found in evening primrose oil. The recommended daily dose for this oil would therefore be 1000 mg.

Side effects: there are no known side effects of taking essential fatty acids at this level.

A multivitamin and mineral supplement

If you are unsure which nutrient to recommend to a patient then it may be more appropriate to recommend a multivitamin supplement. As discussed above, several research trials have shown that good results can be achieved with a multivitamin and mineral supplement called Optivite. Optivite is a multivitamin and mineral supplement which contains large amounts of the B vitamins, magnesium, chromium, vitamin A and vitamin C. While women in the research trials were asked to take six tablets a day it is not recommended that women are advised to take this number of tablets, unless there is adequate medical supervision from a doctor who is experienced in the field of nutritional medicine (six tablets is the equivalent of taking 300 mg vitamin B_6 a day).

Dose: one Optivite tablet a day should be sufficient to correct any vitamin or mineral deficiencies in the majority of women.

Side effects: there should be no side effects at this dosage. If however women take *more* than one tablet a day, they may experience problems such as peripheral neuropathy or diarrhoea.

NB: any patient who is thinking of, or who is actively trying to have a baby should be advised to choose another multivitamin supplement which does not have such a high concentration of vitamin B_6 and vitamin A in it.

Summary

PMS is a debilitating condition and many women seem dissatisfied with current orthodox medical treatment. Nutritional therapy offers an effective, long-term solution for a large percentage of women and this could be offered by the primary care team. Nursing staff could give advice to mild sufferers and dietitians could treat those with severe symptoms. Nutritional therapy should certainly be offered to all women before drug treatment is tried.

Key points – dietary advice for mild PMS sufferers

- Avoid all sugar and foods containing sugar
- Include a wide variety of high fibre foods in the diet
- Eat something every 4 hours – even if it is only some fruit or nuts
- Avoid caffeinated coffee and limit tea to 2–3 cups a day
- Include some meat, fish, eggs, pulses or cheese with the midday *and* evening meals.

Key points – help for severe PMS sufferers

- Patients with severe PMS are often intolerant to yeast or wheat
- There are specific symptoms to look out for which will indicate the presence of a yeast or wheat intolerance
- Dietetic help is required with these patients.

Case studies

Case study 1: a woman with mild PMS

Situation: Alison requested dietary help for her PMS shortly after her second child was born. Her symptoms of irritability and anxiety were lasting for about 8 days out of every month and she felt she was frequently taking it out on the children. In addition, she noticed that she was having more problems with constipation than she had ever had before.

Diet: her diet showed a regular intake of food but most of it was of poor quality with a high reliance on white bread, biscuits and chocolate.

Advice: Alison was given a sugar-free, high fibre diet to which she responded very well. She no longer felt irritable pre-menstrually and her bowel function returned to normal. No nutritional supplement was needed.

Case study 2: a woman with severe PMS

Situation: Sally requested dietary help at the age of 40 for severe PMS. She had tried Femodene but this had made matters worse and a course of evening primrose oil had made no difference. In addition to the severe mood swings she also suffered from insomnia, bad breath and recurrent bouts of vaginal candidosis.

Diet: her diet showed a good intake of fibre but she had rather an addiction to chocolate and a regular intake of sweet biscuits accompanied her cups of coffee throughout the day.

Advice: initially, Sally was advised to cut out all foods containing sugar in her diet and to reduce her caffeine intake. After a month she returned to say this had made no difference and if anything she felt that she was worse. On further questioning it was noted that in the past few weeks Sally had been drinking a lot of wine and had been substituting the chocolate in her diet with cheese. The latter products are both high in yeast and it was decided that Sally was possibly reacting adversely to yeast in her diet. She was therefore given a yeast-free diet to try. This change made a significant difference to Sally's symptoms and she now remains well, without PMS, on a yeast-free diet.

Menus for women with mild PMS

The following menus are free from sugar and are high in fibre. They also include a daily intake of foods which are high in magnesium and the B vitamins.

Day 1

Breakfast
Muesli with milk
1 glass orange juice, diluted

Lunch
Ham salad and jacket potato
Sugar-free yoghurt
Afternoon
Banana
Evening meal
Beef curry with brown rice and courgettes
Toasted tea cake with butter or margarine

Day 2

Breakfast
2 Weetabix with milk
1 slice toast and reduced sugar marmalade
Lunch
Tuna and mayonnaise sandwich
Packet of crisps and an orange
Evening meal
Roast chicken with potatoes, carrots and broccoli
plain, whole milk yoghurt with fruit salad

Day 3

Breakfast
2 slices of granary toast with a poached egg
Lunch
Brown rice salad with onion, tomato, sweet corn, walnuts and raisins
mayonnaise dressing
Banana
Evening meal
Smoked mackerel, peas and new potatoes
Apple pie sweetened with an artificial sweetener

Day 4

Breakfast
Wholemeal muffin with a fruit spread
Glass of orange juice, diluted
Lunch
Cheese on toast
Banana and 60 g mixed nuts

Evening meal
Stir fried vegetables with turkey strips
Brown rice
Stewed rhubarb artificially sweetened and natural yoghurt

Day 5

Breakfast
Cornflakes
1 slice of wholemeal bread with reduced sugar jam
Lunch
Cottage cheese sandwich
and a scotch egg
Evening meal
Gammon steak, jacket potato and coleslaw
Tinned fruit and custard sweetened with an artificial sweetener

Day 6

Breakfast
Porridge
Lunch
Tinned salmon and cucumber sandwich
Packet of crisps
Evening meal
Spaghetti bolognaise with spinach and carrots
Pear

Day 7 (Sunday)

Breakfast
Wholemeal muffin with reduced sugar marmalade
Lunch
Any roast meat with potatoes and vegetables
Fresh fruit salad and cream
Evening meal
Sardines on toast or cream cheese and cucumber sandwiches
A sugar-free fruit yoghurt

References

Abraham G. and Rumley, R. (1987) Role of nutrition in managing the premenstrual tension syndromes. *Journal of Reproductive Medicine*, **32**, 405–422

Biskind, M. S., Biskind, G. R. and Biskind, L. M. (1944) Nutritional deficiency in the etiology of menorrhagia, cystic, mastitis, and premenstrual tension. *Surgical Gynecology and Obstetrics*, **78**, 49

Dalton, K. (1991) *Once a Month*, 5th edn. London: Fontana

Davies, S. and Stewart, A. (1987) *Nutritional Medicine*, edited by A. Stanway. London: Pan Books

Facchinetti, F., Borella, P., Sances, G. *et al.* (1991) Oral magnesium successfully relieves pre-menstrual mood changes. *Journal of Obstetrics and Gynecology*, **78**, 177–181

Freeman, E., Rickels, K., Sondheimer, S. *et al.* (1990) Ineffectiveness of progesterone suppository treatment for premenstrual syndrome. *Journal of the American Medical Association*, **264**, 349–353

Leather, A. T., Holland, E. F. N., Andrews, G. D. and Studd, J. W. W. (1993) A study of the referral patterns and therapeutic experiences of 100 women attending a specialist pre-menstrual syndrome clinic. *Journal of the Royal Society of Medicine*, **86**, 199–201

Sherwood, R. A., Rocks, B. F., Stewart, A. *et al.* (1986) Magnesium and the premenstrual syndrome. *Annals of Clinical Biochemistry*, **23**, 667–670

Stewart, A. (1987) Clinical and biochemical effects of nutritional supplementation on the pre-menstrual syndrome. *Journal of Reproductive Medicine*, **32**, 435–441

Stewart, A., Tooley, S. and Stewart, M. (1991) The effect of a nutritional programme on premenstrual syndrome: a retrospective analysis. *Journal of the Research Council for Complementary Medicine*, **5**, 8–11

Further reading

Stewart, A., Stewart, M., Tooley, S. *et al.* (1992) Pre-menstrual syndrome: is there a basis for a holistic approach? *Maternal and Child Health – The Journal of Family Medicine*, **17**, 86–88

Stewart, M. (1992) *Beat PMT through Diet*. London: Vermilion

Chapter 3
Recurrent vaginal thrush

Introduction

Vaginal thrush or vaginal candidiasis as it is more correctly called, is one of the most common infections seen in general practice and it is estimated that 75% of women suffer at least one episode during their life. The infection, which is usually caused by the yeast *Candida albicans*, produces unpleasant symptoms including inflammation of the vaginal mucosa, severe irritation, a curdy, off-white discharge and sometimes a sensation of burning pain. Most women will only experience candidiasis once or twice in their life and will find that treatment with a local or systemic antifungal agent is effective. Unfortunately, however, there are a number of women who suffer with chronic, recurrent candidiasis, often recurring during the week before menstruation; this condition can be difficult to treat even with systemic antifungal drugs. Many nutritionists now believe that diet therapy can play a useful role in managing recurrent vaginal thrush and therefore the following chapter has been included to describe the dietary advice that should be given to women with this condition.

The incidence and development of vaginal candidiasis

Under normal, healthy conditions *Candida albicans* can be found colonizing the vagina in about 10% of pre-menopausal women and this increases to 30% in pregnant women. For these women the yeast appears to exist quite happily in a non-pathogenic state and does not cause any unwanted symptoms. For some women, however, the yeast can change and develop into a pathogenic form, where it produces the symptoms described above. The patient is then described as having vaginal candidiasis (Figure 3.1). Factors which are believed to influence the development of this pathological state include certain

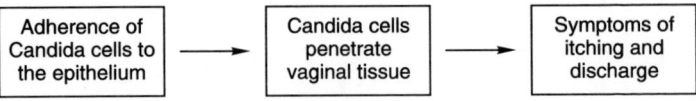

Figure 3.1 The development of vaginal candidiasis

drugs such as cytotoxic drugs, radiotherapy, several metabolic disorders including diabetes, Cushing's disease, Addison's disease and hypo- or hyperthyroidism. AIDS, leukaemia and anaemia which weaken the immune system are also associated with the development of vaginal candidiasis (Scudamore and Allcorn, 1992).

Why is recurrent thrush common in some women and not others?

While many women will experience the occasional episode of vaginal thrush at some time during their lives, there is a group of women who suffer from repeated, chronic vaginal yeast infections and the reasons put forward for this are many and sometimes complex. One theory is that these women are constantly being re-infected by another source, possibly their own gut or from an infected sexual partner. However, practical studies show that reducing intestinal levels of *C. albicans*, or treating male partners does not, unfortunately, have any effect on preventing the recurrence of vaginal thrush in women and therefore this theory is not thought to be very plausible (Working Group of the British Society for Medical Mycology, 1995). Scientists therefore believe that women with recurrent thrush are probably experiencing a relapse of the same infection and the fact that identical strains of the yeast can be isolated after each infectious episode, supports this theory.

Inadequate treatment

One explanation for why some women experience a relapse of the same infection may be that their medical treatment has been inadequate. *Candida* has the potential to be an invasive organism and while topical antifungal creams and pessaries may treat any surface infection, there may be yeast cells which have penetrated deeper into the vaginal tissues which remain untreated. Cells which are not treated may recolonize the vaginal surface again in the future especially if the immune system is compromised in any way.

A poor immune response

While inadequate treatment may play a part in this condition, most clinicians feel that the most likely reason for the recurrence in some women is an impaired immune response to *Candida*. Patients with recurrent vaginal infections rarely have a serious immunological deficiency, but there is some evidence to support the idea that they may have a specific decrease in cellular immunity to *Candida* (Granger, 1992).

Factors associated with vaginal candidiasis

Although there is no evidence to suggest that women with recurrent vaginal candidiasis are more exposed to these precipitating factors than other women, it is useful to be aware of the following conditions which can make women more susceptible to a *Candida* infection:

- Antibiotics
- Oral contraceptives and other hormonal preparations
- Pregnancy
- Diabetes
- Dietary deficiencies
- Clothing and sanitary protection
- Cytotoxic and immunosuppressive drugs.

Antibiotics

A course of antibiotics will sometimes destroy some of the more beneficial bacteria which are present in the bowel and vagina, which help to keep the growth of *Candida* under control. As a result, after a course of antibiotics the growth of *Candida* may go unchecked and diarrhoea and vaginal thrush may develop. This does not happen to all women but is likely to happen to those who are susceptible to vaginal thrush. Some antibiotics appear to be worse than others and broad-spectrum antibiotics have been commonly implicated in the past.

Oral contraceptives and hormones

The Pill has for many years been considered as a positive risk factor for vaginal candidiasis and many patients come off the Pill for this reason. Recent studies, however, suggest that there is no correlation between the use of oral contraceptives and vaginal candidiasis.

Research

Fiona Davidson published the results of her study in 1985 in which the presence of genital candidiasis and contraceptive usage was recorded in over 1300 women at three genitourinary clinics across the country. At the end of the study she found 28% of women had vaginal candidiasis but this was not associated with oral contraceptive use.

Some researchers, however, while acknowledging that progestogen-only contraceptives do not cause a rise in *Candida* colonization, are certain that the oestrogen component of the pill is positively associated with candidiasis (Odds, 1988). If this is true, it could have significant implications for older women who are given oestrogen replacement therapy.

Pregnancy

Vaginal yeast counts are higher in pregnant women when compared with non-pregnant women and studies show that this is particularly so in the third trimester. Hormonal changes are probably responsible for this as the count falls sharply during the puerperium.

Iron deficiency

Several studies have found that an iron deficiency can increase a person's susceptibility to *Candida* infections (Reed, 1992) and this has been my clinical experience also. The immune system is unable to function properly if there is an inadequate store of iron in the body and therefore the infection is likely to persist. Women with recurrent thrush who are suspected of having an iron deficiency should have a serum ferritin test carried out at the beginning of their treatment to check their iron status. (This is a more sensitive test for iron than a full blood count.)

Zinc deficiency

Zinc status can also affect the body's ability to make a full immune response and a mild zinc deficiency has been associated with recurrent vaginal candidiasis (Edman *et al.*, 1986). This should therefore be considered if all other tests have proved normal.

A high intake of sugar

There is some preliminary evidence to suggest that a woman's nutritional intake may have some effect on her risk of vaginal candidiasis (Reed, 1992).

Many clinicians have found that their patients are helped when they remove most of the refined sugar (sucrose) from their diet and, although there is very little published work in this area, where it has been formally evaluated, the results have been very good (Horowitz, 1984). Helping women to reduce the intake of sugar in their diet is therefore worth trying and practical help for this will be given in more detail in the section on dietary advice.

Diabetes

Patients with diabetes mellitus are known to be more at risk of developing a *Candida* infection than people without it and if a patient is backwards and fowards to the doctor with a *Candida* infection it could be that they have an undiagnosed diabetic condition. Conversely, poor control of blood sugar levels in a diabetic may lead to a recurrent *Candida* infection.

Hygiene and clothing

Tight synthetic clothing can create a moist, warm environment in which *Candida* can thrive and women should be advised to wear cotton underwear, stockings rather than tights and loose fitting trousers rather than tight jeans. Hot baths and perfumed soaps are not advisable.

Cytotoxic and immunosuppressive drugs

These drugs taken over a long period of time can depress the immune system and patients undergoing this therapy can become increasingly susceptible to infections including vaginal candidiasis. Similarly, women suffering from AIDS whose immune system is compromised, may be more likely to suffer with recurrent vaginitis.

Medical treatment

Treatment of an acute infection

Most women who consult their doctor with an acute infection are prescribed a topical preparation of an antifungal drug such as nystatin or an imidazole, for example clotrimazole or ketoconazole. These are available as creams or pessaries and all have a low relapse rate. If this does not succeed in eradicating an infection, an oral antifungal drug such as fluconazole, itraconazole or nystatin may be tried.

Treatment of chronic or recurrent infections

Drug therapy can provide symptomatic relief for women with chronic infections but is often unable to eradicate the infection completely. When symptoms keep recurring women find that they either become reliant on their GP prescribing more antifungal drugs each time or that they learn to put up with the symptoms. These women should check whether they have any underlying factors that could be causing their infection to persist, such as the long-term use of antibiotics or the possibility that they may have diabetes, but if these factors can be eliminated – and usually they can – a nutritional approach to managing the infection can be helpful and should be considered.

A nutritional approach

A nutritional approach can be very effective in treating recurrent vaginal candidiasis, especially where other treatments have failed. The Working Group of the British Society for Medical Mycology (1995) recently acknowledged this in their paper on the management of genital candidiasis, in which they reported, 'Patients with recurrent candidiasis often resort to home remedies, such as vaginal yoghurt douches or special diets and there is no doubt that some women derive some benefit from them'.

A nutritional approach aims to help women in two ways:

- Firstly, it aims to improve the functioning of the immune system by increasing the intake of essential nutrients in the diet.
- Secondly, it aims to reduce the growth of the yeast by restricting the intake of sugar in the diet on which the yeast appears to thrive and use as its main substrate.

The diet, which is free from refined sugar and which includes a high intake of fresh fruit and vegetables and a moderate amount of protein, provides the immune system with a high concentration of essential vitamins and minerals. It is a balanced, healthy diet that all women and their families can benefit from and there is nothing particularly difficult about it.

Practical dietary advice for women with recurrent thrush

1 First of all women should be asked about their sugar intake and if this is high they should be advised to reduce it. This involves avoiding cakes, biscuits, desserts containing sugar, chocolate, fizzy drinks, jams, syrups, cereal bars and of course any sugar added to hot drinks. (Small amounts

of sugar found in tinned vegetables, soups or pickles are not harmful and these foods do not need to be avoided.)

2 Women should eat plenty of fresh fruit instead of biscuits and cakes and should choose natural yoghurt rather than fruit yoghurts.

3 Fruit juices should also be avoided as they contain very high concentrations of natural sugars which can aggravate a yeast infection.

4 Women should be advised to choose bread and cereals which are high in fibre, for example brown rice and wholewheat pasta, as these are good sources of B vitamins, iron and magnesium. These are essential nutrients for the health of the immune system.

5 Finally, women should include a good source of iron in their diet each day for example, some red meat, pulses, sardines, eggs or green leafy vegetables.

After a month of following the diet most women should feel that their symptoms are much better. If they are not they should continue to follow the diet for another month and then consult their doctor for further advice.

Live yoghurt is recommended by some practitioners as a douche but there have been no studies to evaluate this therapy so it is not possible for this book to recommend it. Similarly, some books written more generally on the subject of *Candida* infections recommend that dairy products are reduced in the diet. I, however, have not found this to be necessary in the treatment of vaginal *Candida* infections.

Food list

Foods to avoid	Foods to eat plenty of
Sugar	Fruit
Sweetened cereals – e.g. Sugar Puffs	Vegetables
Cakes	Nuts
Biscuits	Brown rice
Sweets	Wholemeal or granary bread
Ice cream	Pulses
White bread and white flour products	Fish
Alcoholic drinks	Eggs
Fizzy drinks	Meat

Summary

Some women can experience recurrent thrush for many months or years and although drug therapy can be used to control the symptoms, it often seems unable to cure the infection altogether. Simple dietary advice should therefore be given to help eradicate this infection. The aim of the advice should be to encourage women to have a nutrient rich diet which will help their immune system to function more efficiently and to avoid any foods which contain added sugar. This could help to resolve the infection within a month.

Key points for giving dietary advice

- Check if the patient is suffering from an iron deficiency by measuring her serum ferritin levels
- Suggest all sugar and sugar containing foods are avoided
- Ensure the patient is eating plenty of high fibre foods
- Advise patients not to drink pure fruit juices, unless they are diluted
- Ask a dietitian to check that there is sufficient iron in the diet to meet the daily requirements
- Recommend that alcohol is avoided or only drunk very occasionally and in moderation.

Case study

Suzanne was 21 years old and was studying languages at university. During the Easter holidays she decided to visit her GP again to ask if there was anything else that could be done about the frequent episodes of thrush that had been plaguing her all term.

Suzanne had been prescribed numerous courses of vaginal pessaries, creams and also a 2-week course of an oral antifungal drug but still the infection persisted. Her GP referred her for a dietary assessment where she was found to be eating an unhealthy diet with lots of chocolate and few fresh vegetables or fruit. Suzanne was persuaded to give up her daily bar of chocolate along with other foods in her diet which contained large amounts of sugar and she was sent to the practice nurse for a serum ferritin test. The results showed that her serum ferritin level was very low: 3 μg/l (normal range 14–148 μg/l) for women (Thomas, 1994) and so she was started on a course of iron tablets. (Her haemoglobin incidentally, was normal.)

Her vaginal thrush cleared up within a fortnight and after 6 months she returned to say she had had no recurrence of any of her symptoms.

Suggested menus for women with recurrent thrush

Day 1

Breakfast
High fibre cereal
Lunch
Granary bread sandwich with cheese and tomato
Packet of peanuts, apple
Evening meal
Shepherds pie
Broccoli, carrots
Natural live yoghurt and tinned pears in their own juice

or
Breakfast
High fibre cereal
Lunch
Wholemeal bread roll with tuna fish and salad
Packet of crisps, orange
Evening meal
Lentil curry
Brown rice and cabbage
Wholewheat crackers and cream cheese

Day 2

Breakfast
High fibre cereal
Lunch
Brown bread sandwich with egg and cress
Diet yoghurt and handful of nuts
Evening meal
Lasagne made with wholewheat pasta
Green salad
Melon and grapes

Day 3

Breakfast
High fibre cereal
Lunch
Jacket potato with chicken mayonnaise filling
Apple
Evening meal
Pork chop
Parsnips, courgettes, sweetcorn
Roast potatoes
Natural live yoghurt and banana

Day 4

Breakfast
High fibre cereal
Lunch
Brown rice salad including spring onion, tuna fish, tomato, sweetcorn and green beans
Peach and banana
Evening meal
Mushroom and bacon omelette
Jacket potato
Green salad
Cheese and wholewheat crackers

Day 5

Breakfast
High fibre cereal
Lunch
Vegetable soup, 2 slices of granary bread
and a piece of cheese
Evening meal
Ham salad
Jacket potato
Stewed fruit and custard sweetened artificially

Day 6

Breakfast
High fibre cereal

Lunch
Bacon, lettuce and tomato sandwich
Pear
Evening meal
Wholewheat pasta shells in a white sauce with tuna, garlic and mushrooms
Broccoli
Diet yoghurt

Day 7 (Sunday)

Breakfast
High fibre cereal
Lunch
Roast meat or vegetarian meal
Vegetables
Fruit salad with cream or yoghurt
Evening meal
2 toasted wholemeal muffins with reduced sugar jam or fruit spread.
Sugar-free fromage frais

References

Davidson, F. (1985) The pill does not cause 'thrush.' *British Journal of Obstetrics and Gynaecology*, **92**, 1265–1266

Edman, J., Sobel, J., Taylor, M. L. *et al.* (1986). Zinc status in women with recurrent vulvovaginal candidiasis. *American Journal of Obstetrics and Gynecology*, **155**, 1082–1085

Granger, S. E. (1992) The aetiology and pathogenesis of vaginal candidosis: an update. *British Journal of Clinical Practice*, **46**, 258–259

Horowitz, B. J., Edelstein, S. W. and Lipman, L. (1984) Sugar chromatography studies in recurrent *Candida vulvovaginitis. Journal of Reproductive Medicine*, **29**, 441

Odds, F. C. (1988) *Candida and Candidosis. A Review and Bibliography*. London: Bailliere Tindall

Reed, B.D. (1992) Risk factors for Candida vulvovaginitis. *Obstetrical and Gynecological Survey*, **47**, 551–560

Scudamore, J. and Allcorn, R. J. (1992). The treatment of acute and chronic vaginal candidosis. *British Journal of Clinical Practice*, **46**, 260–263

Thomas, B. (ed.) (1994) Appendix 2. In: *Manual of Dietetic Practice*, 2nd edn. Oxford: Blackwell Scientific Publications

Working Group of the British Society for Medical Mycology (1995) Management of genital candidiasis. *British Medical Journal*, **310**, 1241–1244

Chapter 4
Women and cardiovascular disease

Introduction

Cardiovascular disease kills one in four women each year and yet little publicity is given to this area of women's health. Men rather than women have been the target of healthy heart campaigns over the past few years, while concerns about breast and cervical cancer have tended to dominate women's health.

However, the publication of a report in 1994 by the National Forum for Coronary Heart Disease, called *Coronary heart disease: are women special?* has helped to put women and heart disease nearer the top of the health agenda.

The main reason that women have not been targeted until now is because coronary heart disease (CHD) develops much later on in a woman's life than in men, about a decade later to be precise, and therefore it is a less sensational condition for them. For example, in 1988 only 66 women died from CHD in England and Wales before the age of 64 compared with 242 men, according to figures published by the World Health Organization. In Scotland the figures were similar with 111 women dying prematurely compared with 320 men.

Women enjoy a relatively low risk of cardiovascular disease when they are young because of the high levels of oestrogen present in their blood. However, when oestrogen begins to decline around the time of the menopause the incidence of heart disease increases dramatically and by the age of 65 men and women show an equal vulnerability to coronary events (Jackson, 1994).

Over the next 25 years the population of post-menopausal women will increase and this will inevitably mean that the number of women affected by cardiovascular disease will also increase. To cope with this clinical demand effectively we need to identify and be clear about any gender differences that exist: for example, whether men and women have different symptoms when they first present with the disease and whether certain risk factors are more important to women. Given this information we should be able to manage the condition more effectively in women.

The following chapter looks at how CHD presents in women, which risk factors are important and the priorities to consider when giving dietary advice. There are also sections on giving advice to women who have had a heart attack and to elderly women.

The incidence of CHD in the UK

Heart disease is still the commonest cause of death in British men and women, despite the fact that deaths from CHD have been falling in men and women since the 1970s. Mortality rates have fallen quite dramatically in younger age groups but there has been little change in the number of deaths occurring in men and women who are between the ages of 55 and 64 (Gregory *et al.*, 1990).

Until the menopause women enjoy significantly less cardiovascular disease than men but after this their mortality figures increase significantly and by the age of 65 they share the same risk as men. The symptoms of CHD are therefore seen most frequently in women who have just retired or in more elderly women; and as the elderly population continues to grow, so too does the problem of cardiovascular disease.

The Clinical presentation of CHD in women

Cardiologists have recently discovered that when women first present with symptoms of heart disease, their clinical presentation is usually different to that seen in men (Jackson, 1994). Here are some of the differences:

- Heart disease usually becomes clinically evident about 5–10 years later in women.
- Women are more likely to present with angina then with an infarction.
- Women are more likely to have diabetes, hypertension and heart failure when they present with coronary artery disease.
- Women who do present with an infarction, often have a more eventful recovery course with a greater risk of death, recurrent infarction or stroke afterwards.

Genetic make up

A person's genetic make up plays a large part in determining how susceptible they are to CHD and although lifestyle factors are important in the development of the disease, the genetic blue print that a person starts out with is, in most cases, the most powerful determining factor. For example, in the USA it is estimated that 5% of families account for about 50% of the coronary deaths that occur before the age of 55 (Myers *et al.*, 1990).

A person's genetic make up is thought to play a significant role in their cholesterol metabolism. For example, some patients will absorb up to 90% of the cholesterol from their diet while others will only absorb 20%. This genetic difference helps to explain why some people appear to be able to eat a very rich diet and enjoy a very low cholesterol level, while others, such as those who have an inherited hypercholesterolaemic condition, often have persistently high cholesterol levels despite following a very low fat diet.

In the future it is possible that with the help of genetic screening we will be able to identify those individuals who are most at risk from CHD. If this happened it could change how we give dietary advice, for example instead of giving out dietary advice to everyone, health professionals could spend more time with those individuals who were most at risk and perhaps most importantly, be able to give advice earlier, before any irreversible damage was done.

Risk factors for coronary heart disease

Several risk factors have been established for CHD and patients are now screened for these in general practice and in the work place. Patients with a family history of heart disease are especially keen to know what their risk level is and how they can reduce it. Smoking, hypertension, and a raised serum cholesterol level, are currently thought to be the main risk factors, but two other factors – a high serum fibrinogen level and an increased platelet size – are also thought to be predicators of coronary disease and may be screened for in the future (Figure 4.1).

Women have up until now been screened and advised about these risk factors in the same way as men despite the fact that the majority of research into risk factors has only been conducted on men. Today, cardiologists are suggesting that men and women may have slightly different risk factors and as a consequence may need to be treated slightly differently.

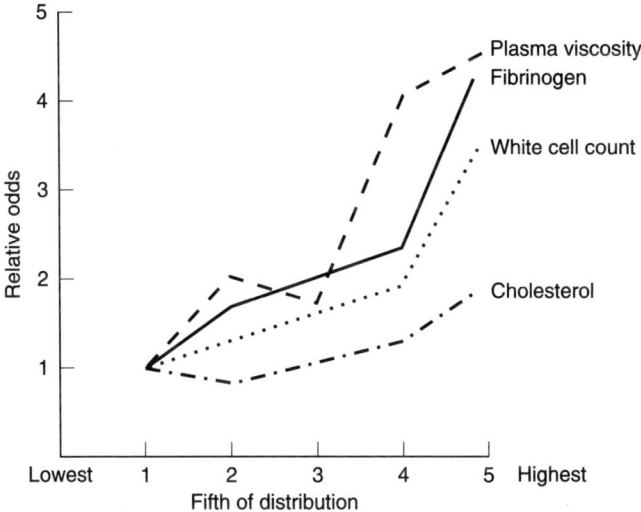

Figure 4.1 MRC risk of coronary heart disease in relation to various haemostatic factors and cholesterol (reproduced with permission)

Risk factors in women

Cholesterol

It is widely recognized that there is a direct relationship between total serum cholesterol levels in middle-aged men and the risk of developing CHD. What is not so clear, however, is the relationship between serum cholesterol levels and CHD in women.

Research: observational studies
Observational studies which have included women suggest that the relationship between total serum cholesterol and CHD is much weaker in women than it is in men and this was recently highlighted in a Scottish study, in which 15 000 adults were followed up for 15 years.

The researchers found that women were much more likely to have a higher serum cholesterol level than men but were at significantly less risk from CHD. While there was a general trend for mortality rates to increase in women as their cholesterol levels increased, their risk of mortality from CHD was still lower than that of men even when their plasma cholesterol levels were high. Thus women in the *top* quintile for cholesterol had a lower

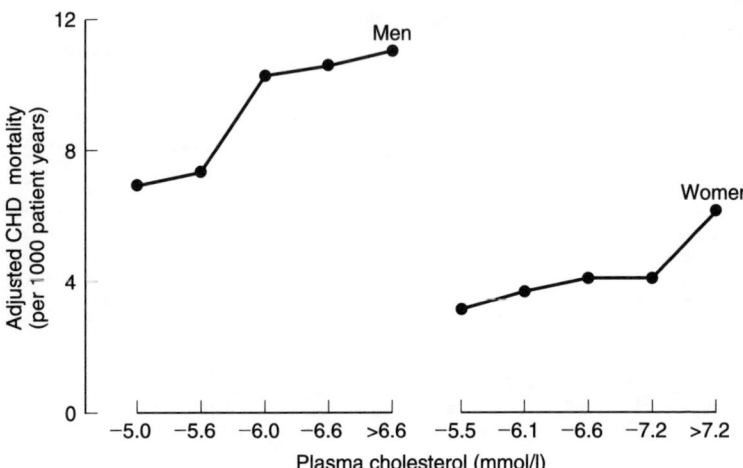

Figure 4.2 Male and female mortality from CHD to quintile of plasma cholesterol. (Reproduced from Isles *et al.* (1992) *The Lancet*, i, 702–706 by kind permission of the Editor)

coronary mortality than men in the *bottom* quintile (Isles *et al.*, 1992) (Figure 4.2).

Intervention studies
At present no study has demonstrated that lowering moderate to high cholesterol levels in otherwise healthy women has any effect on their mortality. Only studies that have been carried out on women with established cardiovascular disease have shown that there are benefits from lowering cholesterol levels.

Lipoproteins

The four lipoproteins which transport cholesterol around the body can give additional information about a person's coronary risk. For women high density lipoproteins (HDL cholesterol), which are inversely associated with a person's risk of heart disease, are currently thought to be a more accurate predictor of coronary risk in women, compared with low density lipoprotein (LDL cholesterol) levels. Therefore, if a woman has a high level of HDL cholesterol present in her plasma, it is unlikely that she will go on to develop CHD.

Triglycerides

Triglycerides are another lipid in the blood and high levels are thought to be strongly associated with CHD in women – more so than in men. In addition the normal range for triglycerides in women is thought to be lower than it is for men (Table 4.1).

Table 4.1   Recommended serum lipid levels for women

Lipid	Desirable range for women (mmol/l)
LDL	1.7–5.62★
HDL	0.89–2.05★
Triglycerides	0.1–0.76★★
Cholesterol	2.5–5.5 (desirable)

Thomas, B. (1994) *Manual of Dietetics*, Blackwell Science Ltd
★This value is slightly higher in women than it is in men.
★★This value is significantly lower in women than it is in men.

Hypertension

High blood pressure is an independent risk factor and anyone developing it will increase their risk of developing heart disease and cerebral vascular disease. Hypertension is frequently found in women who have developed CHD and cardiologists believe that it could be an even stronger predictor of cardiovascular disease in women than it is in men (Jackson, 1994). Drug treatment of hypertension has been shown to be effective at reducing the risk of cerebrovascular disease, but there is no firm evidence yet to show that it reduces the incidence of CHD.

Smoking

Cigarette smoking has, for a long time been associated with an increased risk of cardiovascular disease and the decline in smoking over the last two decades, in men *and* women, may account for the overall fall in CHD in both sexes.

Smoking is thought to be harmful for a number of reasons:

- Carbon monoxide, present in inhaled smoke reduces the level of oxygen which is available to the heart.
- Chemicals found in cigarette smoke may damage cell membranes and DNA.
- Nicotine and carbon monoxide may increase the tendency for blood to clot.
- Fibrinogen levels are, on average, higher in smokers than in non-smokers.

Obesity

Obesity, particularly central obesity, is known to be an independent risk factor for CHD and some scientists feel that the hip to waist ratio, i.e. the degree of *central* obesity present, may be a more sensitive risk factor for CHD than body mass index (BMI). This is discussed further in Chapter 1.

Fibrinogen levels

It has been argued that the risk factors described above – smoking, blood pressure and cholesterol – can only explain some of the incidence of heart disease in men and women and therefore researchers have continued to look for other risk factors than may help the medical profession to understand why some people become ill.

Recently, research (unfortunately conducted only on men) has found that fibrinogen levels are strongly predictive of CHD. Fibrinogen is a plasma

Table 4.2   The relative value of risk factors for CHD in men and women

Risk factors	Men	Women
Total cholesterol	+++	+
HDL cholesterol	+	++
LDL cholesterol	+++	+
Triglycerides	+	++
Hypertension	+	++
Smoking	+++	+++
Diabetes	+	+++
Fibrinogen	+++	?

+++ Very predictive; ++ fairly predictive; + mildly predictive protein involved in the clotting process and several studies have shown that there is a strong independent association between high fibrinogen levels and the progression of peripheral vascular disease (Ernst, 1990). Of particular interest to those working in general practice is the observation that higher fibrinogen levels have been found in people who smoke.

Some doctors would like to see patients being screened for high fibrinogen levels in the same way that they are screened for cholesterol. The relative risk factors for CHD in men and women are summarized in Table 4.2.

The pathogenesis of coronary heart disease

The pathogenesis of CHD is thought to occur in three separate stages:

- Stage one: arterial injury
- Stage two: atherosclerosis
- Stage three: formation of a thrombus (thrombosis).

There is strong evidence that diet can play a part at all three stages.

Arterial damage

Arterial damage is currently thought to be caused by lipids such as cholesterol and triglycerides which, in their oxidized form become highly reactive chemical products which are readily taken up by the arterial wall. Smoking and hypertension are also thought to be involved in the process of arterial damage.

The role of diet

Antioxidants such as vitamins A, C and E have an important part to play in preventing the oxidation of cholesterol and other lipids and there is now much evidence to suggest that people who have a diet which is rich in these vitamins suffer much less from atherosclerosis than those whose diets are poor in these vitamins.

Atherosclerosis

Atherosclerosis is the accumulation of cholesterol and other lipids within the arterial wall and this leads to a narrowing of the arterial lumen and damage to the arterial surface. LDL cholesterol, in its oxidized form, is thought to be particularly damaging and involved with the process of atherosclerosis. Serum cholesterol levels can be lowered by dietary or drug means and this seems to minimize the process of atherosclerosis in midde-aged men. The effects of lowering cholesterol levels in middle-aged women, however, are not known and many cardiologists question whether this is necessary in women who are otherwise healthy.

Recent evidence suggests that women are able to tolerate much higher serum cholesterol levels than men without experiencing the same high coronary mortality rates (Isles *et al.*, 1992) and more research with women is clearly needed to evaluate this area.

The role of diet
Until there is further information on women and serum cholesterol levels women should be advised to eat a balanced varied diet.

Formation of a thrombus

The formation of a thrombus or blood clot in a coronary artery which has been narrowed by atherosclerosis can result in a myocardial infarction. Patients who smoke tend to have higher concentrations of clotting factors in their blood and this of course makes them more susceptible to thrombosis.

The role of diet
A regular intake of oily fish is thought to be important in inhibiting thrombus formation. Various groups of people around the world, including the Innuits of Greenland and the fishing communities in Japan consume large amounts of oily fish each day and experience very low rates of cardiovascular disease. The Innuits can eat up to 500 g of whale meat a day which is the equivalent of 14 g of the n–3 series of polyunsaturated fatty acids. This is in sharp contrast to the UK diet where the average intake of n–3 fatty acids is 1.6 g/day. As a community the Innuits have a lower platelet count and experience longer bleeding times when compared to other communities in that geographical region and this is all thought to be due to their high consumption of fish.

Patients can, however, certainly gain similar benefits from eating much lower intakes of fish. In the Netherlands for instance, communities who consume 30 g of oily fish each day enjoy a 50% reduction in the incidence of heart disease compared to other areas of the Netherlands where very little fish is eaten.

Giving dietary advice to women who are at risk of developing cardiovascular disease

The following section discusses the major topics that usually arise when giving dietary advice to women who are concerned about the prevention of heart disease and should help you to answer any questions that may be put to you. For example, questions such as 'Can I eat nuts?' or 'What are trans fatty acids?' or 'Do I have to give up butter?'. Many patients have an overall idea of what they should be doing but sometimes need help with the details of their diet and this section should provide most of the answers.

Specific areas of a patient's diet

Saturated fat intake
Women should aim for a moderate reduction in saturated fat.

- Sunflower, corn oil, olive oil or soya oils should be used in cooking rather than butter or hard margarine.
- Fatty meat and processed meat, e.g. sausages, hamburgers, pork pies etc. should only be eaten occasionally.
- Shop-bought cakes and biscuits contain a considerable amount of saturated fat and so where time permits women should make their own using a good quality polyunsaturated margarine.
- Hard cheese should be restricted to 100 g a week.

Vegetable oils
Oils from vegetables, nuts and seeds are important as they provide a person with several essential fatty acids which the body cannot manufacture itself. These oils are also a good source of vitamin E which is an important antioxidant and known to protect the body from CHD. In culinary terms, vegetable oils also help to increase the palatability of the diet.

Sunflower, corn oil or soya oils can be used for making salad dressings, stir frys, brushing lean meat to be grilled or potatoes to be roasted and for frying meat and vegetables before they are used in a casserole. All varieties of nuts should be encouraged as they are a healthy snack food which contain high concentrations of essential fatty acids and minerals.

Most fruit and vegetables are low in natural oils with the exception of the avocado pear: this fruit is high in essential fatty acids and vitamin E and so it is quite suitable for anyone concerned about their cholesterol level.

Fish oils

There are several ways in which the oils present in fish are thought to protect the heart and blood vessels (Pritchard, 1995). First, fish oils have a beneficial effect on serum lipids: they help to lower triglyceride levels and also to raise levels of high density lipoproteins, which are associated with protecting the body against heart disease. In addition to this, fish oils are believed to improve the vasodilatory properties of blood vessels and may inhibit the clotting process.

Eating oily fish appears to have a very beneficial effect on patients who have had a myocardial infarction (MI); in one study in which 2000 survivors of an MI were followed up, those who were told to eat 300 g of oily fish a week had a much lower mortality rate in the 2-year follow-up period compared with other patients who had been given different dietary advice (Burr *et al.*, 1989).

In practice people should be encouraged to eat oily fish several times a week. Tinned sardines, tuna, pilchards and mackerel are not expensive and make good sandwich fillings or can be grilled on toast. For a more substantial meal, herrings, whole mackerel, trout or sardines are delicious with fresh vegetables, chips cooked in sunflower oil or a brown rice salad.

Cholesterol

Cholesterol in the *diet* as opposed to cholesterol in the *body*, is not considered to be harmful any more, particularly if the saturated fat content of the diet is low.

In practice patients should be allowed to eat normal quantities of liver, kidney, eggs and shell fish in their diet.

Antioxidants

The antioxidant vitamins – vitamin E, vitamin C, vitamin A and carotene – are found in fruit and vegetables and are believed to make an important contribution towards reducing the risk of heart disease in men and women. They are believed to do this by protecting polyunsaturated fatty acids from oxidation. Low plasma levels of these vitamins have been linked with a higher risk of angina pectoris in men (Riemersma *et al.*, 1991).

The Mediterranean diet is rich in fruit and vegetables and this is thought to be the main reason for the low rates of heart disease in countries such as Italy, France and Greece.

In practice, today the World Health Organisation recommends that everyone eats 500 g of fruit and vegetables each day. This is roughly equivalent to five portions, for example a banana, an apple, a serving of cabbage, peas and carrots each day. This advice is also being advocated by those interested in the prevention of cancer.

Trans fatty acids

Trans fatty acids are formed when vegetable oils are hydrogenated (hardened) during an industrial process and made into margarine. They are also formed when vegetable oils are heated to a high temperature, for instance in frying. Some scientists feel that these are harmful substances which can cause heart disease, however, so far there is little evidence to prove this.

Fibre intake

Some studies have demonstrated that dietary fibre may have a role in helping to lower cholesterol levels. Soluble fibre, which is found in oats and pulses, is reported to be particularly effective at lowering LDL cholesterol levels while keeping HDL cholesterol levels high and so it is frequently recommended. Wheat bran on the other hand does not seem to have any affect on cholesterol levels.

In practice patients with a significantly raised cholesterol level should be encouraged to include some oats in their diet each day. The easiest way to do this is to have an oat-based cereal for breakfast, for example muesli or porridge. Pulses which can be recommended to most people are peas, green beans or baked beans, while chick peas, cannelloni beans, pinto beans and mung beans may be recommended to more adventurous patients. Pulses can easily be incorporated into vegetable lasagnes, vegetable or meat casseroles and rice dishes.

Most pulses can now be bought ready soaked in a tin which working women will find more convenient.

Vitamin E

It is widely recognized that certain European countries have a high saturated fat intake and yet enjoy a relatively low rate of coronary heart disease among their people. Numerous dietary reasons have been put forward to explain this paradox but, at present, the most likely reason is that they have much higher intakes of vitamin E than we do in the UK.

Vitamin E is found mainly in the vegetable oils that Mediterranean households use so liberally in their cooking and it is also found in vegetables such as carrots, tomatoes, asparagus, broccoli, green peppers and sweetcorn.

In practice people should not be discouraged from using vegetable oils such as sunflower, soya and corn oils as these are excellent sources of vitamin E. If people were encouraged to eat more vegetables and salad foods with their main meal this would also increase their intake of vitamin E.

Facts about individual foods

Red meat
Many individuals who are at a high risk of developing CHD are often told not to eat any red meat. This is not necessary, however, and is not, I believe, the best advice, especially for women. Certainly a person's diet will benefit from substituting some of their red meat intake for fish and chicken and dishes using pulses but cutting red meat out altogether is unlikely to benefit female patients. Lean meat does not have a high saturated fat content and is an excellent source of iron, zinc and the B vitamins. These nutrients are needed daily by women and by including some red meat in their diet two to three times a week, they can easily avoid becoming low in these nutrients.

Coffee
There has been much controversy over the issue of coffee and heart disease but recent evidence suggests that there is very little additional risk from drinking instant or filter coffee on a regular basis.

Olive oil
Olive oil is high in monounsaturated fatty acids and these, like polyunsaturated fatty acids appear to have a neutral or possibly even beneficial effect on blood lipid levels. Some scientists believe that monounsaturated oils such as olive oil may be safer than polyunsaturated oils because they are less susceptible to oxidation in the body, but this has not yet been proved.

Olive oil is a time-honoured oil which has been used for centuries in the Mediterranean where the incidence of heart disease is low. The combination of using olive oil rather than hard saturated fats to cook with together with a high intake of fruit, vegetables and wine in that region is certainly thought to have a protective effect. Patients may like to use this type of oil in cooking, although it is more expensive than other vegetable oils.

Butter
All foods, including butter, should be seen in the context of the whole diet and women who enjoy butter and who otherwise have a healthy diet should not feel that they have to give it up. Butter is best kept for use on toast, scones or tea cakes where it is really going to be tested. Margarine on the other hand can be used in sandwiches and in baking.

Eggs

Traditionally eggs have been restricted on the diets of patients with heart disease because they are high in cholesterol. This is no longer necessary however, as *dietary* cholesterol, such as the cholesterol found in eggs, has only a very small effect on *serum* cholesterol. It is the saturated fat content of the diet rather than the cholesterol content of the diet that has the greatest effect on serum cholesterol and so foods such as eggs, shell fish and liver which are high in cholesterol but which do not contain large amounts of saturated fat, can be eaten in normal quantities.

Alcohol

Women who drink alcohol in moderation are more likely to enjoy a lower risk of coronary heart disease than non-drinkers according to most epidemiological studies (Razay *et al.*, 1992). This is thought to be because a moderate intake of alcohol is associated with lower triglyceride and insulin levels and higher HDL cholesterol levels in women. Drinking within the guidelines laid down by the Health Education Authority can therefore be recommended to women.

Dietary advice for special groups

Dietary advice for those who have had a myocardial infarction

Women who have had a myocardial infarction should be given advice as soon as they are well enough to receive information. By changing their diet they can minimize the chances of having another attack and for many it is a psychological boost to feel that there is something positive that they can do to help themselves. They are usually very motivated patients.

The best advice to give this group, according to limited research, is to encourage a diet high in oily fish. In the DART trial in which over 2000 men recovering from an MI were given three different types of dietary advice, a high intake of oily fish was associated with a significant reduction in mortality compared with those who were not given this advice and the authors concluded that a modest intake of oily fish, i.e. two to three portions per week may reduce mortality in men who are recovering from an MI (Burr *et al.*, 1989).

Until such a trial is carried out on women it is difficult to know whether fish can convey the same benefits for them as well. However, we know that a high fish intake in many Scandinavian and polar communities has a beneficial effect on cardiac health and so it seems sensible at present to include women in this advice.

In practice, therefore, women should be encouraged to choose tuna, sardines, tinned salmon or pilchards for their sandwich fillings rather than ham or cheese, and should consider cooking trout, mackerel, herrings or salmon as an alternative to meat for their main meal two or three times a week.

Advice for the elderly patient

High cholesterol levels in the elderly population appear to be associated with an increased risk of CHD in the same way that they are in younger people. However, at this time in life, dietary advice should not be too strict and should be tailored to the situation.

Many elderly people have physical or mental disabilities to contend with and food and meal times become highlights in their day, which should be respected. After 50 years of eating cheese on toast four nights a week, roasting potatoes in lard or having double cream on fruit salad they are unlikely to want to change and who can blame them for this. Personally, I feel time is much better spent checking that patients are eating a *balanced* diet, including sufficient protein and vitamins, rather than trying to persuade them to lower their fat intake.

Some elderly patients who take on board the current healthy eating message can get over enthusiastic about their low fat diet and care should be taken to check that they do not lose too much weight through this. Similarly some elderly people can include too much fibre in their diet particularly if they are using processed bran. This can cause them to suffer from excessive wind, and abdominal pain and should be discouraged. They should be advised to have more fruit and vegetables if they are concerned about their fibre intake.

In conclusion, elderly patients should be enjoying their food at this time in their life and ways in which this enjoyment can be increased, rather than curtailed should be the main priority when discussing their diet with them.

Preventing heart disease in the future: nutrition during pregnancy

The prevention of coronary heart disease has, until now, centred on changing the dietary behaviour of young and middle-aged adults. In the future we may see this change with a greater emphasis placed on the importance of good nutrition at the very beginning of life – during pregnancy.

Professor David Barker and his team at the MRC unit in Southampton have found that babies who are small at birth are more likely to develop coronary heart disease, hypertension, strokes and diabetes during their adult life and this is thought to be due to an inadequate delivery of nutrients to the fetus during pregnancy (Barker, 1990). In an interesting study involving several hundred men and women who were born at the beginning of this century, his team found that death rates from coronary heart disease fell in adults as their birth weights increased. In addition to this, he has found that other body measurements at birth could also be linked to the development of certain coronary risk factors later in life. Initially his research focused on men but, recently, similar results have been found in women (Fall *et al.*, 1995).

As a background to this Professor Barker believes that an adequate delivery of nutrients to the fetus is essential for ensuring that normal development takes place and has suggested that research should be directed more towards the intrauterine environment rather than the environment in childhood, such as housing, family income and diet (Barker, 1990).

Summary

Coronary heart disease does not affect many women before the menopause but is commonly seen in older women. Although women appear to be less affected by some of the main risk factors, such as a high cholesterol level, the main pathology of CHD is the same as in men and therefore women too should benefit from some dietary advice.

In the past, the emphasis of dietary advice has centred around recommending a low fat intake, but today this advice should be adjusted as certain oils, such as those found in nuts, fish and vegetables are now recognized as being very beneficial. In addition to this, fruit and vegetables have also gained a higher priority in the diet as they offer considerable protection against CHD.

Women should therefore be encouraged to have a balanced diet which includes a variety of polyunsaturated oils and plenty of fruit and vegetables.

Key points about risk factors

- The same coronary risk factors apply to women as they do to men, but to different degrees

- Total cholesterol is only weakly associated with CHD in women

- Diabetes and smoking are strongly associated with CHD in women

- Oestrogen protects most women from CHD until the menopause

- More research is needed to establish whether there are other risk factors for women.

Key points about diet

- Patients should reduce their intake of foods which contain a lot of saturated fat in them such as pork pies, fatty meat, hard cheese, full fat soft cheeses, pastries, biscuits and some cakes

- Other sources of fat found in vegetable oils, nuts, and oily fish do not have to be reduced in the diet as they are polyunsaturated fats

- Patients should be encouraged to eat a lot of fresh fruit and vegetables, ideally three fruits and two portions of vegetables each day

- Where possible they should also be encouraged to eat fish, oily or white, three or more times a week

- Adequate amounts of starchy foods such as bread, cereals, potatoes, rice and pasta should be eaten with each meal so that high fat snacks such as chocolate, biscuits, crisps and pastries are not needed in between meals.

Case studies

Case study 1: a high serum cholesterol level

Carol is 45 years old and has made an appointment to discuss her cholesterol level which is 7.05 mmol/l. She has no clinical symptoms of heart disease, has a reasonably healthy lifestyle playing squash twice a week, and does not think there is any premature heart disease in her family.

Her diet is good:

Breakfast	Cereal or toast
	Polyunsaturated margarine/semi-skimmed milk
Lunch	Cheese, egg or ham salad with a brown roll
	yoghurt or chocolate biscuit
Evening	Roast or casseroled meat most days
	Pizza once a week
	Lots of fresh vegetables
	Jelly, tinned fruit, ice-cream or cheesecake for dessert.

Advice

It should be explained to Carol that high cholesterol levels are only weakly associated with heart disease in women and that she should only be concerned if there are other risk factors present, such as a low HDL cholesterol level or a high triglyceride level present. (If necessary, these blood tests should also be carried out to reassure her.)

While discussing her diet you could suggest the following.

- Have some fish either at lunch or in the evening, twice a week
- Have some fresh fruit or fruit juice daily.

Case study 2: a woman with angina

Dorothy is 60 years old. She has severe angina and is on the waiting list for a coronary bypass operation. She is overweight with a BMI of 30 and her blood pressure is high. Her cholesterol level is within the normal range but her triglyceride levels are raised.

Her diet is as follows:

Breakfast	Tea with 1 tsp. sugar and plain biscuit
Lunch	Meat in some form (shepherd's pie, lasagne, roast)
	White fish once a week
	1 vegetable
	Potatoes
Evening	Sandwich or something on toast
	and a piece of cake
Supper	Hot chocolate and 1 plain biscuit

Advice

Dorothy's weight and high blood pressure are significant risk factors. The priority for Dorothy is to lose some weight, especially if she is suffering from central obesity, i.e. excess weight around her abdomen, as this is strongly associated with CHD in women.

If Dorothy is able to lose some weight her blood pressure and triglyceride levels should fall and of course it should mean that she is in a better condition for her operation.

To do this she should be encouraged to cut out all biscuits, cakes and anything else that she is having that contains any sugar. This relatively simple instruction helps a lot of people to lose weight and does not mean that they continually have to feel hungry. Instead she should eat more fruit, cereals, yoghurts and nuts.

In addition to this the type of bread she is eating could be checked. Some people find that their weight loss is more successful when they change from white to brown bread.

Patients who have a medical condition such as Dorothy's, which improves with weight loss, are very likely to be successful and certainly monitoring their blood pressure regularly and showing that there is a downward trend can be as good an incentive for someone as watching kilograms or pounds disappear.

Menus for a healthy heart

These menus are based on the current thinking that a moderate intake of polyunsaturated oils is fine for men and women as long as they are having a good intake of fruit and vegetables as well. A regular intake of fish is thought to be particularly beneficial and so several meals including white and oily fish have been included.

Day 1

Breakfast
Porridge
Fruit juice
Lunch
Tuna mayonnaise sandwich
Orange and banana
Evening meal
Lean roast beef
Green beans, cabbage, parsnips
Boiled potatoes
*Home-made apple pie and custard

Day 2

Breakfast
Muesli
Fruit juice
Lunch
Chicken and salad sandwich
Pear and grapes
Evening meal
Potato and cashew nut curry
Brown rice

Broccoli, carrots
Yoghurt and banana

Day 3

Breakfast
Porridge
Fruit juice
Lunch
Cottage cheese and raisin sandwich
2 tomatoes
A packet of peanuts
A banana
Evening meal
Grilled mackerel
New potatoes
Peas, cauliflower
*Home-made carrot cake

Day 4

Breakfast
Muesli
Fruit juice
Lunch
Tuna and tomato sandwich
Apple and banana
Cereal bar
Evening meal
Shepherd's pie using lean minced lamb
Cabbage, baked beans
Tangerine
Crackers and low fat cream cheese

Day 5

Breakfast
Porridge
Fruit juice
Lunch
Prawn and mayonnaise sandwich
Raw carrot

Banana and 2 plums
Evening meal
Vegetable lasagne
Green salad
*Home-made lemon sponge pudding with plain yoghurt

Day 6

Breakfast
Muesli with banana or apple chopped up on it
Lunch
Brown rice salad with nuts, raisins, sweetcorn, cold chicken and mayonnaise
Evening meal
Fish pie, peas and courgettes
Fruit crumble and custard

Day 7 (Sunday)

Breakfast
Porridge
Lunch
Roast meat or vegetarian dish
Vegetables
Fruit sorbet
Evening meal
Egg sandwiches
Scones with jam
Fruit
*Home-made puddings and cakes should be made using a polyunsaturated margarine.

CHD questionnaire

Ten questions which can be used quickly to assess the quality of a patient's diet and determine if they are at risk from CHD.

Part A

1 Do you eat a piece of fresh fruit every day?
2 Do you eat vegetables (other than potatoes) every day?

Part B

1 Do you use a vegetable oil in cooking?
2 Do you eat oily fish, e.g. tuna, sardines, mackerel twice a week?
3 Do you have semi-skimmed or skimmed milk at home?

Part C

1 Do you eat biscuits most days?
2 Do you eat chocolate most days?
3 Do you eat sausages or beefburgers more than once a week?
4 Do you eat more than 4 oz hard cheese a week?

Interpretation of the results

Ideal response
A patient who answers 'yes' to all questions in parts A and B, and 'no' to all questions in part C has a very good diet and their risk of CHD should be small.

Acceptable response
A patient who answers 'yes' to the questions in part A, 'yes' to at least one question in part B and 'no' to half the questions in part C will, generally, have an acceptable diet.

Unacceptable response
A patient who answers 'no' to either of the questions in part A and 'yes' to most of the questions in part C has a diet which is, in the long term likely to cause significant health problems.

Author's note: the above interpretation is only intended as a guide.

Part A is, in my opinion, the most important aspect of the diet and for a diet to be acceptable patients must answer 'yes' to both these questions. It is also desirable for patients to answer 'yes' to Part B but not imperative. Part C reveals the negative aspects of a patient's diet and if there are many positive responses to these questions this suggests a very processed diet which is associated with an increased risk of CHD.

References

Barker, D. J. P. (1990) The fetal and infant origins of adult disease. *British Medical Journal*, **301**, 1111

Burr, M. L., Holliday, R. M., Gibert. J. F. *et al.* (1989) Effects of changes in fat, fish, and fibre intakes in death and myocardial re-infarction: diet and re-infarction trial (DART). *Lancet*, ii, 757–761

Ernst, E. (1990) Plasma fibrinogen – an independent cardiovascular risk factor. *Journal of Internal Medicine*, **227**, 365–372

Fall, C. H. D., Osmond, C., Barker, D. J. P. *et al.* (1995) Fetal and infant growth and cardiovascular risk factors in women. *British Medical Journal*, **310**, 428–431

Gregory, J. *et al.* (1990) *The Dietary and Nutritional Survey of British Adults.* London: HMSO

Isles, C., Hole, D. J., Hawthorne, V. M. and Lever, A. F. (1992) Relation between coronary risk and coronary mortality in women of the Renfrew and Paisley survey: comparison with men. *Lancet*, i, 702–706

Jackson, G. (1994) Coronary artery disease and women. *British Medical Journal*, **309**, 555–556

Myers, H. R. *et al.* (1990) Parental history is an independant risk factor for coronary heart disease. The Framingham Study. *American Heart Journal*, **120**, 963–969

National Forum for Coronary Heart Disease (1994) Coronary heart disease: are women special?

Prichard. B. N. (1995) Fish oils and cardiovascular disease. *British Medical Journal*, **310**, 819–820

Razay, G., Heaton, K. W., Bolton, C. H. *et al.* (1992) Alcohol consumption and its relation to cardiovascular risk factors in British women. *British Medical Journal*, **304**, 80–82

Riemersma, R. A., Wood, D. A., MacIntyre, C. C. A. (1991) Risk of angina pectoris and plasma concentrations of vitamins A, C and E and carotene. *Lancet*, **337** (8732), 1–5

Thomas, B. (ed.) (1994) Appendix 2. In: *Manual of Dietetic Practice* second edition. Oxford: Blackwell Scientific Publications

World Health Organization (1989) World Health Statistics Annual. Geneva: WHO

Further reading

Barker, D. J. P. (1994) *Mothers, Babies and Disease in Later Life.* London: BMJ Books

Chapter 5

Osteoporosis

Introduction

Osteoporosis is a condition in which a person's bone mass gradually decreases with age and leaves them more susceptible to fractures. There is no change in the composition of bone, as occurs in osteomalacia, but simply a net loss and as a result the bones affected become fragile and break with only a minimum amount of trauma. To help with identifying the causes, osteoporosis has been classified in to two types:

- type 1: post-menopausal osteoporosis
- type 2: senile osteoporosis.

Type 1 occurs, as its name suggests, predominantly in women around the time of the menopause and is characterized by vertebral and Colles (wrist) fractures. Type 2 occurs later, from 65 years onwards and can occur in men or women, although again there is a higher incidence in women. It is characterized by fractures of the hips.

Osteoporosis has been called the 'silent disease' because bone loss can occur over many years, without the patient ever being aware of it. Bone is a living tissue and throughout life it is continually being deposited and then reabsorbed back into the circulation. Throughout childhood and adolescence, bone *deposition* is the dominant process in the body and by about the age of 30 years bone mass has reached its peak. Shortly afterwards, however, the process is reversed and *resorption* of bone takes place at a greater rate than bone deposition and the result is that bones gradually become less dense and more fragile with age. The long bones of the body become thinner but the bones present in the skull do not seem to change.

Gradual bone loss with age is a universal phenomenon that can be observed in all races and both sexes, regardless of geographical location or

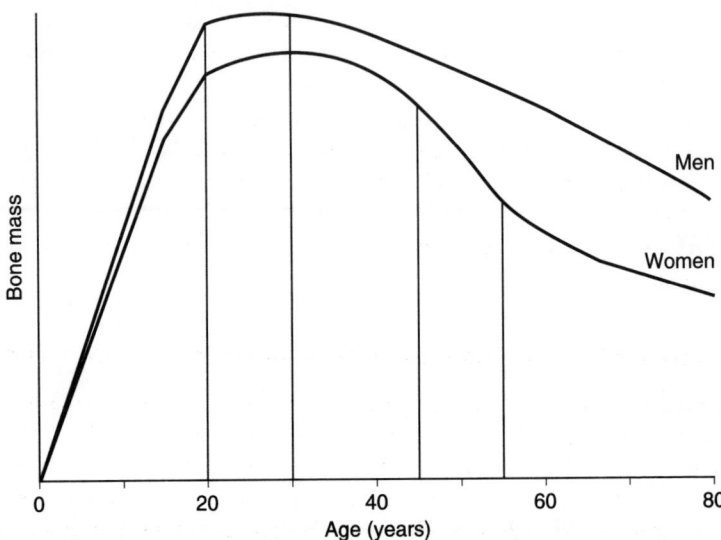

Figure 5.1 Change in bone mass with age. (Reproduced from Clunie (1994) *British Journal of Hospital Medicine*, by kind permission)

economic status (Figure 5.1). The incidence of osteoporosis, however, is much higher among people living in developing nations and this has led some scientists to suggest that a sedentary lifestyle may be responsible for the higher incidence.

Why are women more vulnerable to osteoporosis?

Women are more vulnerable to osteoporosis than men for three reasons:

- Women do not achieve such a high peak bone mass by the time they are 30, compared with men.
- The process of bone loss starts at an earlier age in women.
- The rate of loss is greater: approximately 1% a year compared with 0.3% a year in men.

This accelerated bone loss occurs around the time of the female menopause: bone loss at the time of the menopause is significant for many women; a lack of oestrogen at this time in their life leads to an accelerated loss of bone, particularly trabecular bone, which is found predominantly in the spinal column. As a consequence, vertebral fractures are frequently seen in this age group and one estimation suggests that as many as 7% of post-menopausal women in the UK, suffer with vertebral fractures (Cooper *et al.*, 1991).

This chapter looks at the environmental and medical factors which increase the risk of developing osteoporosis; and then at the importance of calcium throughout the life cycle. At the end of the chapter is a section on prevention of osteoporotic fractures in the elderly and a questionnaire which can be used in the clinic to screen for a low calcium intake in adults or children.

Factors which increase the risk of developing osteoporosis

Genetic disposition plays a large part in the development of osteoporosis and this was highlighted by some research which found that daughters of mothers with osteoporosis have lower bone mass density measurements than daughters of mothers who were not affected by this condition (Seeman *et al.*, 1989). However, some women will be more at risk than others because of their lifestyle (Table 5.1).

Table 5.1   Factors which have a negative effect on bone density

- A poor calcium intake in childhood and adolescence
- Inactivity at all ages
- Smoking
- A low body weight
- Exercise-induced amenorrhoea

Poor calcium intake in childhood and adolescence

The bone mass which is achieved in the first two decades of life, plays a major part in determining the bone mass of adults later on and therefore there is great interest in which factors affect the development of bone mass in children. Along with regular exercise, it is essential that children have an adequate intake of calcium. Calcium, together with vitamin D, has for a long time been recognized as an important nutrient for the health and development of the skeleton, but the amount that children require is a controversial area; requirements may actually be higher than originally thought and this will be discussed in more detail in Section 4 which focuses on calcium requirements throughout the life cycle.

Inactivity

Low levels of physical activity lead to a fall in bone density and patients who are forced to curtail their activity over a long period of time because of a chronic illness must be considered as being at risk. Regular exercise is important for all age groups: in children exercise is associated with achieving maximum bone density and in post-menopausal women it is associated with minimizing bone loss. Weight-bearing exercise increases bone density more effectively than other types of exercise, so walking, running and racket sports for example, are more beneficial for this condition than swimming.

Smoking

Smoking accelerates post-menopausal bone loss (Krall and Dawson-Hughes, 1991) and in case control studies smoking has been identified as a risk factor for vertebral fractures (Aloia *et al.*, 1985). All attempts should be made to persuade women to stop smoking *before* the menopause so that their chances of a vertebral fracture or hip fracture later on are reduced.

Low body weight

Women whose body weight falls below a BMI of around 20 usually develop amenorrhoea or irregular periods. This is usually accompanied by low levels of oestrogen and can lead to a loss of bone. Women who are underweight for a long period of time are more at risk of developing osteoporosis than average or overweight women.

Exercise-induced amenorrhoea

While moderate exercise has a beneficial effect on bone density and is to be encouraged, intensive exercise and training can have just the opposite effect. Strenuous aerobic exercise undertaken by professional or even serious amateur athletes, can have an affect on the hypothalamic – pituitary – gonadal axis and this causes a reduction in the amount of oestrogen and progestrogen which is released from the ovaries. In adolescent girls this leads to the delay of the menarche and irregular, or even an absence of, periods. The long-term consequences of low oestrogen levels in the body are rather serious so far as the skeleton is concerned. Female athletes can suffer from brittle bones in the same way that post-menopausal women can, and stress fractures become more common, particularly in athletes with menstrual irregularities. If amenorrhoea is only for a short period, i.e. 6 months, then bone loss can be easily

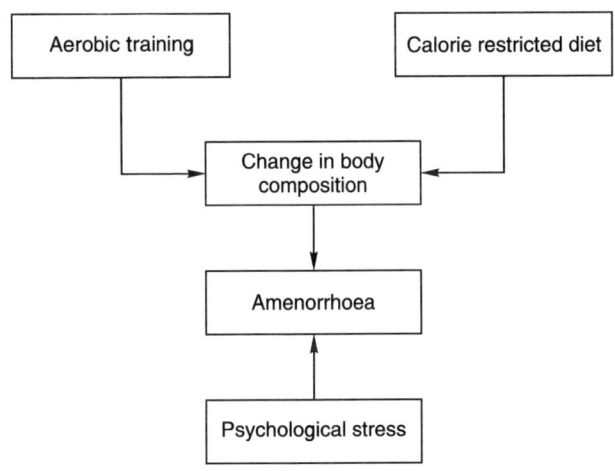

Figure 5.2 Adverse effects of intensive training. (Reproduced from Wolman (1994)
British Medical Journal, by kind permission)

regained. However, if periods are absent for several years the loss may be irreversible and calcium and oestrogen supplements may be needed to prevent premature osteoporosis.

Athletic amenorrhoea is a relatively recent problem; it was first noticed in the late 1970s and reflects the more punishing training regimens that have recently been introduced for athletes. Today up to half of women who are first class ballerinas, runners or rowers are believed to be amenorrhoeic (Wolman, 1994).

The cause of amenorrhoea in athletes is related both to the intensity of training *and* to the level of calorie restriction in the diet. The reduction in body fat that occurs with training and dieting is thought to be a critical factor in the development of amenorrhoea (Figure 5.2).

Advice for athletes
- Any woman who has been amenorrhoeic for 6 months should have a medical assessment.
- Women with amenorrhoea should discuss the feasibility of reducing their training schedule with their trainer.
- All women undergoing intensive physical training should be referred to a dietitian for an assessment of their calcium and energy intake.

Medical conditions associated with osteoporosis

The medical conditions associated with an increased risk of osteoporosis are listed in Table 5.2.

Table 5.2   Conditions associated with osteoporosis

Metabolic and hormonal
Ovarian failure
Amenorrhoea
Pregnancy
Hyperthyroidism
Cushing's syndrome
Corticosteroid therapy
Chronic liver disease
Chronic renal disease
Malabsorption

Inflammatory, neoplastic and mechanical
Rheumatoid or Inflammatory arthritis
Myeloma
Low mechanical stress: paraplegia and immobility

Reproduced from: Clunie (1994), *British Journal of Hospital Medicine* by kind permission

The importance of calcium throughout the life cycle

The prevention of osteoporosis is a life-long process and the following section looks at the calcium requirements for children, adults, and the elderly.

Calcium for children and adolescents

Children and adolescents needs to take in slightly more calcium than they need if skeletal growth is to be at an optimum level. In other words they need to be in a state of positive calcium balance.

Growth of the skeleton during the first two decades of life shows two peaks: one during infancy when an infant will double his or her skeletal mass during the first year and the other during adolescence. Large amounts of calcium are retained by the body at these stages (Table 5.3).

Table 5.3 Retention of calcium

Age	Calcium (mg/day)
Early infancy	160
Childhood	70–150
Adolescence	250 for girls, 300 for boys

Dietary Reference Values for Food Energy and Nutrients for the United Kingdom (1991) London: HMSO

Calcium requirements
Calcium requirements have been set according to the amount of calcium children need at each stage of their growth and an additional amount has been recommended to allow for the fact that not all of the calcium in the diet will be absorbed (Table 5.4).

Table 5.4 Calcium requirements in children and adolescents

Age	Reference nutrient intake (mg/day)	Food equivalent
0–12 months	525	Normal intake of breast or formula milk
1–3 years	350	284 ml cow's milk and 2 slices bread
4–6 years	450	284 ml cow's milk, 3 slices bread and 2 vegetables
7–10 years	550	As above plus 28 g cheese or yoghurt
11–18 years, male	1000	568 ml milk, 3 slices bread and 28 g cheese or yoghurt
11–18 years, female	800	426 ml milk, 3 slices bread and 28 g cheese or yoghurt

HMSO, 1991.

Are children getting enough calcium?

According to dietary surveys, most children appear to be getting sufficient calcium to meet the Government's current recommendations. In 1986 the Department of Health collected data on the diets of more than 3000 British school children aged 10–11 and 14–15 and found that children in the younger age group had good calcium intakes between 700 mg and 800 mg. Girls in the 14–15 age group, however, did not have adequate calcium intakes. Their intake of calcium remained at around 700 mg which is 100 mg short of their daily requirement, and the main reason for this appeared to be because their intake of milk and puddings fell, instead of increasing (Department of Health, 1989).

Milk and dairy foods remain the main source of calcium in our diet, and unless there is a medical reason for a young person not being able to tolerate them, they should be encouraged in the diets of teenagers who have high calcium requirements. If girls are not keen on drinking milk they should be encouraged to have a generous amount on their cereal each morning and a yoghurt each day which, in calcium terms is equivalent to having 200 ml milk. They should also be encouraged to have hard cheese in their sandwiches 2–3 times a week, as well as cottage cheese as hard cheese is a much richer source of calcium.

Calcium supplements for children

Following the publication of a study, which showed calcium supplements could increase bone density by as much as 5% in children (Johnston *et al.*, 1992), there has been renewed interest in whether calcium should be prescribed for this age group. The above study, carried out in the USA on children whose diets already met the government recommendations for calcium, has challenged whether the current requirements are sufficient to allow children to achieve their *peak* bone mass and whether if children were given even more calcium they could achieve further increases in bone mass. Certain studies have suggested that only a small increase in peak bone mass in the population could lead to a large reduction in the number of fractures that occur later in life and so the above study could have important clinical implications.

Further research is needed in this area: we need to know whether children are capable of 'catch up' skeletal growth and if they are, for how long this opportunity exists. Similarly, we need to find out if the recommended reference nutrient intakes, set by the government, really are adequate. For now parents should not be advised to rush out and buy calcium supplements but should be educated on which foods are good sources of calcium.

Calcium requirements during the menopause

Accelerated bone loss lasts for about 5 years around the time of the menopause and taking additional calcium in the diet may or may not reduce the
amount of bone which is lost during this phase (Department of Health,
1991). There is no general medical consensus on this issue as research studies
have shown conflicting results and women should be aware of this. Women
entering this new phase in life, however, will naturally want to seek advice
about their diet and in particular want to know about their calcium intake.
They should be advised to have an *adequate* intake of calcium but should be
aware that it is debatable whether very high intakes are more beneficial.
Women of this age are recommended to have 700 mg calcium a day, which
is equal to:

- 426 ml milk, 2 slices of bread *and* a small portion of cheese, or yoghurt
  or some tinned fish with bones in it (e.g. salmon, pilchards or
  sardines).

For many women this may seem like a large intake of milk to consume
each day. Many women, particularly those watching their weight, will tend
to drink low calorie fruit drinks or black coffee throughout the day and will
also avoid hard cheese. These women are therefore a good group to target in
Well Women clinics where a few simple dietary questions can quickly evaluate whether they are getting sufficient calcium or not. As well as dairy
products some nuts, fish and vegetables are also good sources of calcium
(Table 5.5).

Table 5.5   Other non-dairy sources of calcium

Muesli
Dried figs, dried apricots, dates, raisins
Rhubarb, blackberries
Broccoli, cabbage, turnip, carrots
Spinach, baked beans, water cress
Haddock, prawns, shrimps
Almonds, brazil nuts

Calcium supplements
The benefits of taking a calcium supplement during the menopause are debatable. Some studies show mild improvements in bone mass when calcium
supplements are taken, while others have found no change at all. Certainly

patients with osteoporosis do not seem to show any improvements in their condition when they are treated with calcium alone. The fall in oestrogen at this time in women, causing the sudden acceleration in bone loss probably overrides any benefits that additional calcium, in supplemental form can make. Patients who are being treated with oestrogen, however, may benefit from taking a calcium supplement.

Other dietary considerations for menopausal women

High alcohol intake

Alcohol accelerates bone loss and if it is consumed in large amounts patients may suffer from significant bone loss. Alcoholics are also more prone to falls and this will tend to increase their chances of sustaining a fracture.

Caffeine intake

Caffeine increases urinary calcium excretion and at high intakes this may contribute to a negative calcium balance (Heaney and Recker, 1982). If, for example, women are consuming around 10 cups of percolated coffee a day or 15 cups of instant coffee a day, this could potentially have a negative effect on their bone mass and they should be advised to reduce it and find an alternative drink.

Medical treatment for women with osteoporosis

Muscle pains and an aching sensation in bones and joints at the time of the menopause are usually symptoms of osteoporosis, and the treatment that is most commonly used to treat osteoporosis is oestrogen.

Oestrogen replacement therapy

Oestrogen replacement therapy is the choice of treatment used by most doctors and it is usually very effective. Oestrogen will prevent bone loss at any age (Lufkin et al., 1992) and as long as it is being taken the benefits continue. As soon as it is discontinued bone loss begins to accelerate again and so most women are recommended to take it for at least 10–15 years. The use of oestrogen for post-menopausal women is of course a controversial area with many advantages and disadvantages and there are many medical reviews available which discuss the subject in detail.

Dietary advice for the elderly

The incidence of hip fractures increases dramatically after the age of 65 years and current figures suggest that nearly one in four women living until they are 90 years old, will suffer a fractured hip (Law, Wald and Meade, 1991). This places a huge burden upon the health service and accounts for a significant percentage of hospital admissions each year. In an attempt to try to prevent osteoporotic fractures in the elderly there are two preventative measures that those working with the elderly can try: firstly, it is worth giving elderly patients a calcium and vitamin D supplement if they are house bound Secondly, they should be made as stable as possible, to reduce their chances of falling and sustaining a fracture.

Vitamin D and calcium supplements

Offering a daily vitamin D supplement to elderly house-bound patients could be a very inexpensive and simple way of preventing many hip fractures. The elderly are at risk from a vitamin D deficiency as many of them do not get out very much and therefore have little exposure to sunlight. In addition to this, a poor diet and the presence of systemic or renal disease may mean that they are not metabolizing the vitamin very effectively. As a result, secondary hyperparathyroidism can occur in elderly women and this is associated with the development of a low bone density (Khaw *et al.* 1992; Chapuy *et al.*, 1994). This, however, can be corrected by giving supplements of vitamin D and calcium to elderly people who live in nursing homes and the risk of hip fractures and other non-vertebral fractures can be reduced substantially (Chapuy *et al.*, 1994).

Low calcium intakes are not very common in the adult population but may occur among some elderly women who have very small appetites. Calcium supplements are generally very inexpensive and are a small price to pay if it helps to avoid a hospital admission.

Level of supplementation:

- 1–1.2 g of calcium
- 20 μg vitamin D (cholecalciferol)

Increasing a person's stability

It has been observed that many elderly people who have a low bone mineral density do not necessarily develop any fractures and one reason for this may be that some elderly people are much more stable on their feet. Helping the elderly to achieve a better level of general health can be an important way of helping elderly people preserve their stability. For example ensuring that they have regular eye checks so that they maintain good visual acuity, and regular exercise so that they preserve their muscle tone and are able to maintain their balance. Preventing osteoporotic fractures in the elderly is almost certainly about caring for various aspects of a person's mobility, as well as their bone mass.

Summary

Osteoporosis is when a loss of bone mass leads to fractures. It is more common in women and there is a strong genetic factor associated with its incidence. Smoking, inactivity, and a low intake of calcium during childhood are the greatest environmental risk factors associated with osteoporotic fractures and women who are genetically at risk should be especially aware of these factors. An adequate calcium intake throughout life is important in the prevention of osteoporosis, but is particularly important during childhood and adolescence when much of the skeletal mass is being formed. While most children have adequate intakes of calcium it seems that some adolescent girls do not consume sufficient dairy products or other sources of calcium to meet their needs. This group should be targeted in general practice.

Bone loss around the time of the menopause is greater than at any other time during a woman's life and this is due to the falling levels of oestrogen in the body. Calcium supplements at this time are unlikely to reduce bone loss significantly and a more general approach to education may be more beneficial.

The elderly are particularly susceptible to hip fractures and those over 75 years of age who live in a nursing home or who are largely house bound should be recommended to take a vitamin D and calcium supplement.

Key points

- Lifestyle factors account for 20% of the variance in bone mass

- An adequate calcium intake is essential in children and adolescents if they are to achieve their peak bone mass

- Children and adults who are intolerant to dairy products will normally need a calcium supplement   (continued opposite)

(continued)

- Children and adults should be encouraged to participate in regular exercise
- Women should be encouraged to give up smoking before the menopause
- Elderly men and women who do not get out very much may benefit from a vitamin D and calcium supplement.

Case studies

Case study 1: osteoporosis and the menopause

Monica is 45 and is entering the menopause. She is working full time as a computer programmer and has two teenage children.

She is anxious about developing osteoporosis because her mother has suffered from the condition. She knows that calcium is important for a healthy bone structure, but does not know very much else about the condition. She smokes 15 cigarettes a day and shares a bottle of wine at the weekend with her husband.

Her diet is fairly well balanced with cereal for breakfast, a wholemeal sandwich for lunch and chicken or fish usually for her evening meal with plenty of vegetables and either potatoes or brown rice. She loves anything made from chocolate and regularly has a piece of chocolate cake or chocolate mousse for supper. Her intake of milk is about 284–426 ml per day.

Advice: Monica should be reassured that her calcium intake is good. She should however be advised to stop smoking and be encouraged to find some weight-bearing activity to do.

Case study 2: calcium intake in a 10-year-old girl

Georgina had severe colic as a baby which was linked to an intolerance to cow's milk and ever since then she has been unable to tolerate dairy products and has had soya products instead. Her appetite is good: for breakfast she has cereal with soya milk and a slice of toast, for lunch she takes 2 rolls, a piece of cake and a carton of fruit juice and in the evening she eats a variety of foods including pizza without the cheese, spaghetti bolognaise, a meat casserole or a vegetable or meat curry.

She has about 284 ml soya milk a day.

Advice: despite a good appetite it is unlikely that Georgina is getting enough calcium because of her intolerance to dairy products. Her mother should try to buy soya milk which has calcium added to it and her diet should be assessed by a dietitian to find out how much more she may need to take in the form of a supplement.

A questionnaire to screen for calcium deficiency

The following questionnaire is intended for use in the clinic to check quickly whether a child or adult is getting enough calcium. The answers are interpreted below.

1 Do you have 284 ml milk a day?	300 mg
2 Do you eat vegetables every day?	100 mg
3 Do you eat 28 g nuts every day?	80 mg
4 Do you eat a yoghurt every day?	240 mg
5 Do you have 113 g hard cheese a week?	140 mg/day
6 Do you have 3 slices brown or white bread a day?	100 mg

Answers:
a) Yes to all questions = 960 mg calcium.
This is a high intake of calcium that would be adequate for all ages.
b) Yes to most questions (including question 1) will give an intake of about 650–700 mg.
This will be adequate for most age groups *except* 11–18 year olds who really need to be having 426–568 ml milk per day.
c) Yes to only three questions (not including question 1) will give an intake ranging from 280 to 480 mg.
This may be adequate for small children up to six years but not older children, adolescents or adults.

Menus high in calcium for adolescents

Providing 800–1000 mg calcium a day for 11–18 year olds

Day 1

Breakfast
*Cereal with milk
2 slices toast and peanut butter
1 glass fruit juice

Lunch
Ham sandwich
Apple and pear
*56 g almonds
Evening meal
*Mushroom quiche
Coleslaw
Jacket potato
*Yoghurt
Supper
*Milky drink and piece of sponge cake

Day 2

Breakfast
2 slices toast with jam or honey
Glass fruit juice
Lunch
*Cheese and pickle sandwich
Apple and banana
*56 g dried fruit and nut mix
Evening meal
Shepherd's pie
Baked beans
Cabbage
Fruit pie and *custard
Supper
*Milky drink and biscuit

Day 3

Breakfast
*Cereal with milk
2 slices toast with Marmite
Glass fruit juice
Lunch
*Tinned salmon (including bones) sandwich
Apple and orange
*Yoghurt
Evening meal
*Vegetable lasagne

Salad
*Ice cream and tinned fruit
Supper
*Milky drink and biscuit

Day 4

Breakfast
Cereal with milk*
1 slice toast with marmalade or jam
Lunch
Tuna fish sandwich
Banana and scone*
Evening meal
Vegetable* chilli and rice
Yoghurt *and stewed fruit
Supper
Milky drink* and biscuit

Day 5

Breakfast
Cereal with milk*
1 slice toast with jam or marmalade
Lunch
Cottage cheese* salad with nuts* and raisins
Large jacket potato
Fromage frais*
Evening meal
Grilled fish
Chips, peas and carrots
Sponge pudding and custard*
Supper
Milky drink*

Day 6

Breakfast
Scrambled egg
2 slices toast
Lunch
Grated cheese* on a jacket potato

Baked beans*
Evening meal
Stir fried vegetables and prawns*
Brown rice
Banana and custard* or yoghurt*
Supper
Milky drink* and piece of sponge cake*

Day 7

Breakfast
Cereal with milk*
1 slice toast with Marmite
Lunch
Sardines* on 2 slices of toast
Scone* and apple
Evening meal
Roast meat
Potatoes, carrots, sweetcorn and green vegetable (broccoli or spinach)*
Apple pie and ice cream*
Supper
Milky drink* and banana

References

Aloia, J. F., Cohn, S. H., Vaswani, A. *et al.* (1985) Risk factors for post menopausal osteoporosis. *American Journal of Medicine,* **78**, 95–100

Chapuy, M. C., Arlot, M. E., Delmas, P. D. *et al.* (1994) Effect of calcium and cholecalciferol treatment for three years on hip fractures in elderly women. *British Medical Journal,* **308**, 1081–1082

Clunie, G. (1994) Osteoporosis prevention. *British Journal of Hospital Medicine,* **52**, 70–85

Cooper, C., Shah, S., Hand, D. J. *et al.* (1991) Screening for vertebral osteoporosis using individual risk factors. *Osteoporosis International,* **2**, 48–53

Department of Health (1989) *The Diets of British Schoolchildren.* Report on Health and Social Subjects. no. 36, London: HMSO

Department of Health (1991) *Dietary Reference Values for Food Energy and Nutrients for the United Kingdom.* London: HMSO

Heaney, R. P. and Recker, R. R. (1982) Effects of nitrogen, phosphorus and caffeine on calcium balance in women. *Journal of Laboratory and Clinical Medicine,* **99**, 46–55

Johnston, C. C., Miller, J. Z., Slemenda, C. W. *et al.* (1992) Calcium supplementation and increases in bone mineral density in children. *New England Journal of Medicine*, **327**, 82–87

Khaw, K. T., Sneyd, M. J., Compston, J. *et al.* (1992) Bone density, parathyroid hormone and 25 hydroxy vitamin D concentrations in middle aged women. *British Medical Journal*, **305**, 273–276

Krall, E. A. and Dawson-Hughes, B. (1991) Smoking and bone loss among postmenopausal women. *Journal of Bone Mineral Research*, **6**, 331–337

Law, M. R., Wald, N. J. and Meade, T. W. (1991) Strategies for prevention of osteoporosis and hip fractures. *British Medical Journal*, **303**, 453–459

Lufkin, E. G., Wahner, H. W., O'Fallon, W. M. *et al.* (1992) Treatment of postmenopausal osteoporosis with transdermal oestrogen. *Annals of Internal Medicine*, **117**, 1–9

Seeman, E., Hooper, J. L., Bach, L. A. *et al.* (1989) Reduced bone mass in daughters of women with osteoporosis. *New England Journal of Medicine*, **320**, 554–558

Wolman, R. L. (1994) Osteoporosis and exercise. *British Medical Journal*, **309**, 400–403

Chapter 6
Women and cancer

Introduction

Cancer is the clinical name used to describe a process of abnormal cell division which can occur any where in the body at any time in a persons life. If it is allowed to continue, the group of cells which are dividing in an abnormal way form a tumour and this can invade the surrounding tissues causing harm to nearby organs and depriving the healthy cells of essential nutrients.

Fortunately, most cancers are now treatable and doctors working in the field of oncology claim that 50% of cancer patients are now cured completely, and many more are able to live for much longer periods after their diagnosis than they were 10 years ago (Dawson, 1990). This has come about because many new techniques, designed to eradicate the harmful cancer cells, have been pioneered in the last few decades, including chemotherapy, radiotherapy, hormone therapy and now the use of monoclonal antibodies. While this treatment offers much hope to people who have been diagnosed with cancer, actually undergoing the treatment is usually a very traumatic experience and in the future it is hoped that greater information about the causes of cancer will allow a greater emphasis to be placed on prevention.

At present we know that our genetic make up, the environment in which we live, our nutritional intake and our immune system all play a decisive role in determining whether or not we will develop cancer. In this chapter the link between cancer and nutrition will be discussed starting with a look at how cross cultural studies have increased our knowledge, followed by a section on how food can either help to protect us or make us more at risk and then a more in depth look at the role of nutrition in breast cancer and endometrial cancer. The chapter finishes with a look at whether vitamin supplements are of any value in preventing cancer.

The link between cancer and nutrition

Diet is believed to play a significant part in the aetiology of many cancers and some scientists believe that if people made the appropriate changes to their diet they could reduce their risk of cancer by at least one third and possibly by two thirds (Austoker, 1994). This conclusion has come about largely as a result of many crosss cultural observations made by epidemiologists such as Professor Doll, who have found that the incidence of cancer varies greatly across the world. Cancers of the colon and breast, for example, are very common in western developed nations, while cancer of the stomach is more prevalent in Japan and cancer of the liver is common in certain parts of Africa.

There is now strong evidence to suggest that the reason for specific cancers being more prevalent in one geographical region than another is because of the different lifestyles and diets that are found in each region (Doll and Peto, 1981; Rose, Boyar and Wynder, 1986). When people move from an area of low cancer risk to an area of high cancer risk they soon develop the same high risk as the indigenous population adding further evidence to support this theory. A good example of this is the Japanese community: in the 1950s and 1960s many of them migrated to Hawaii and quickly adapted to a more westernized lifstyle on the island. Unfortunately epidemiologists soon observed that these immigrants were developing the same high risk of breast and colonic cancer that people who had been living there all their lives were experiencing and it was therefore concluded that lifestyle rather than genetic predisposition was the primary cause. The Japanese are not the only community to have experienced this and Doll and Peto in their book *The Causes of Cancer* describe other groups of people who have moved from one country to another who have experienced this phenomenon (Doll and Peto, 1981).

Diet has therefore been established as a primary factor in the development of certain cancers, and two theories have been put forward to explain how it may have an effect. Both theories are valid:

1 First, certain foods are believed to provide *protection* against cancer.
2 Secondly, certain foods are believed to make a person more *susceptible* to cancer.

Foods that offer protection against cancer

Fruit and vegetables

A large intake of fruit and vegetables can provide great protection against many cancers, but particularly against cancers of the gastrointestinal tract and the respiratory tract (Austoker, 1994). Fruit and vegetables are rich sources of vitamins A, C, E and carotene and it is thought that these vitamins may be involved in protecting the body against the development of cancer. Vitamins A, C, E and carotene can collectively be described as *antioxidant vitamins*. These act by preventing various chemicals in the body, including dietary fats from undergoing a process of oxidation. The oxidation of dietary fats is thought to produce products which can potentially cause cancer and therefore there is concern among health professionals that this process should be prevented or minimized. Eating a diet high in fruit and vegetables is one way of doing this.

Dietary advice to patients
All patients, and especially those with a family history of cancer, should be encouraged to eat plenty of fresh fruit and vegetables in their diet. The World Health Authority has recommended that five portions of fruit and vegetables should be consumed every day: this is equivalent, for example, to a good sized portion of carrots, cabbage, and courgettes with an evening meal and an apple and banana eaten sometime throughout the day. This is not an unrealistic amount of fruit and vegetables to expect people to eat but many do not achieve this amount on a regular basis.

Another point to remember, is to encourage patients to eat a *wide variety* of fruit and vegetables so that they are sure of obtaining a good intake of all the antioxidant vitamins. Oranges, for example, are a rich source of vitamin C while carrots and apricots are good sources of vitamin A. The following gives a list of fruit and vegetables which are rich sources of the antioxidant vitamins.

Good sources of carotene and vitamin A: apricots, green leafy vegetables, tomatoes and carrots.

Good sources of vitamin C: citrus fruits, bananas, potatoes, peppers, raw cabbage.

Good sources of vitamin E: avocado pears, nuts.

Fibre

Dietary fibre is also believed to be a protective factor against cancer and a low intake in the past has been linked with the development of certain cancers, particularly cancer of the colon. However, most recent research shows conflicting results and the relationship between dietary fibre and cancer of the colon is not clear. A high intake of fibre from fruit and vegetables, as opposed to cereal fibre however, has been shown to be consistently linked with a lower risk of cancer of the colon (Willett, 1989).

Dietary advice to patients
Patients should be encouraged to have five portions of fruit and vegetables each day. Sweetcorn, pulses, bananas, carrots, cabbage, broccoli and peas are particularly good sources of fibre.

Foods that increase the risk of developing cancer

Fat

When epidemiologists have compared patterns of food consumption across the world they have found a strong association between the intake of animal fat and the incidence of breast, ovary, prostate and colon cancer (Rose, Boyar and Wynder, 1986). However, many case control and prospective studies have not supported the idea that a high intake of animal fat necessarily leads to the development of cancer, except in the case of cancer of the colon where there appears to be a definite link (Willett *et al.*, 1990). The flow diagram shown in Figure 6.1 illustrates the role of animal fat as a carcinogen in colonic cancer.

Alcohol

Certain cancers have been directly linked to the overconsumption of alcohol: these are cancers of the mouth, larynx, pharynx, liver and oesophagus. They

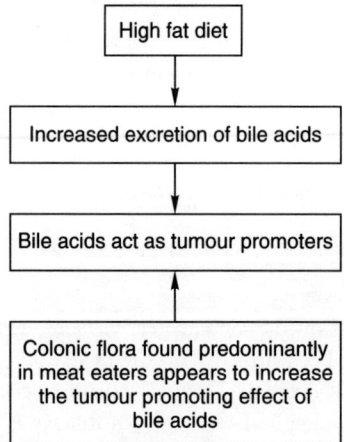

Figure 6.1 A possible mechanism as to how a high fat diet might lead to cancer of the colon.

are not very common cancers but still account for a significant proportion of deaths each year because they tend to be quite difficult to treat.

People who smoke at the same time as drinking heavily, dramatically increase their risk of developing cancer in the head and neck region. The reason for this is not fully known but some scientists feel that alcohol may help to dissolve the cancer-causing substances found in cigarette smoke and help them to enter the body more easily.

Women are recommended by the Health Education Authority to drink less than men because, physiologically, they are less able to cope with large amounts of alcohol. To avoid the cancers described above they should be advised to keep to 14 units a week.

General overnutrition

Overnutrition, leading to obesity, also seems to be a risk factor in the development of certain cancers and seems to play an important role in the development of endometrial and gall bladder cancer in women. Obesity is also a risk factor for breast cancer in post-menopausal women and this will be discussed in more detail later in the chapter.

Breast cancer

Breast cancer is the most common form of cancer among women in the UK making up approximately 20% of all cancer registrations. Each year around 29000 women are diagnosed as having breast cancer and 16000 women die from it (Macmillan Breast Cancer Campaign, 1994). The incidence of breast cancer increases with age: approximately 10 cases per 100000 are diagnosed in women under 30 years, and this increases to 150 cases per 100000 in women aged 50 (Dawson, 1990).

Dietary fat intake and the risk of breast cancer

Women in the UK have a high mortality rate from breast cancer compared with women in other countries (Table 6.1). Epidemiologists such as Richard Doll and Richard Peto have for a long time associated this with differences in our diet and in particular with the differences in our fat intake (Figure 6.2).

When mortality figures for breast cancer are compared with figures for the national consumption of fat, there appears to be a strong relationship between animal fat consumption and the mortality rate from breast cancer (Figure 6.2).

Table 6.1   Mortality rate from breast cancer

Country	Mortality rate/100 000 1964	Mortality rate/100 000 1978
Japan	3.8	5.2
Greece	7.5	14.3
Spain	7.5	14.0
Poland	10.3	14.0
Portugal	12.6	14.5
Finland	13.5	14.9
Italy	15.7	18.5
Norway	16.9	19.1
Austria	17.1	18.7
UK	24.4	27.7

However, despite these cross cultural observations, so far no prospective nor case control study of any reputation has been able to show that there is a clear relationship between either total or saturated fat intake and the risk of breast cancer. This may possibly be because all the research has been carried out in western developed countries where the variation in fat intake is not very great. For example, the lowest intake of fat in the UK is typically around 32% of energy intake and it is possible that the incidence of breast cancer would not change significantly until women reduced this to below 30% of their energy intake. Alternatively, it may be that some other dietary factor is the reason for the significant difference in breast cancer rates between countries and that this has yet to be identified.

Vitamin A and breast cancer

The role of the antioxidant vitamins A, C, E and beta carotene in preventing cancer was discussed at the beginning of this chapter in relation to the prevention of all cancers. Several studies, including a large study of 89 000 women in the USA, have found an inverse relationship between a woman's vitamin A intake and her risk of breast cancer (Hunter *et al.*, 1993). The association, however, only seems to apply to women with very low intakes and therefore only those with a very poor quality diet need to be given advice about including foods containing vitamin A or advice about taking a supplement.

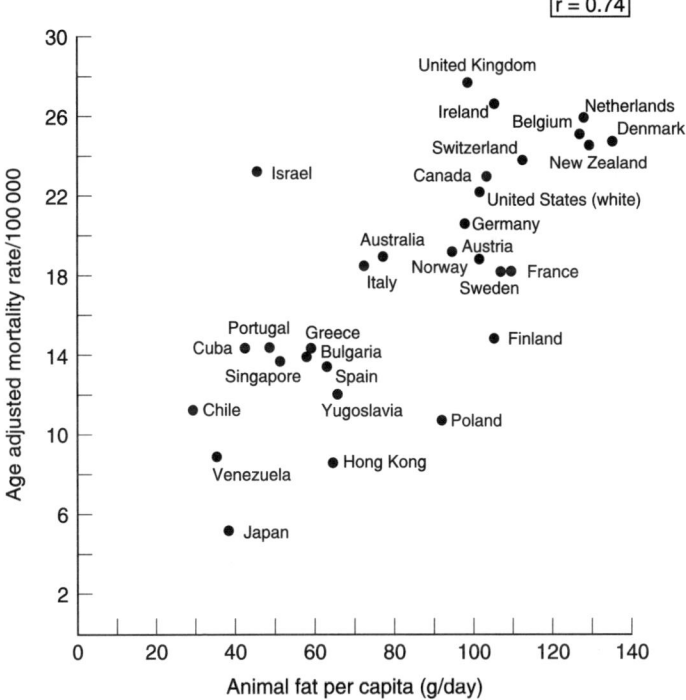

Figure 6.2 Correlation between age-adjusted breast cancer mortality rates for 30 countries and available fat *per capita*. (Reproduced from Rose, Boyar and Wynder (1986) *Cancer*, by kind permission)

Good sources of vitamin A

Vitamin A is found in liver, eggs and dairy products. Carotenoids, which can be converted into vitamin A by the body, are found in vegetable products and fruit. Rich sources of carotene are carrots, spinach, spring greens, water cress, broccoli, tomatoes, apricots and peaches.

Obesity and breast cancer

Overnutrition, leading to obesity, is associated with an increased risk of developing breast cancer in post-menopausal women. Recent research suggests that the type of obesity that women experience may also be important, with women who gain weight predominantly in the *upper* part of the body being more at risk (Schapira *et al.*, 1994). This type of obesity is called *android* obesity and involves weight gain around the abdomen, shoulders and nape of the neck rather than around the buttocks and thighs which is called *gynoid* obesity. People who gain excessive amounts of weight in the upper parts of their body are also more at risk factor of developing cardiovascular illness, diabetes, hypertension and lipid abnormalities; and women who are genetically susceptible to this type of obesity should be encouraged at an early stage in their life to eat sensibly and take regular exercise.

Other non-dietary factors associated with the development of breast cancer

Age at menarche

Girls who start menstruating at an early age are generally more at risk of developing breast cancer (Henderson and Bernstein, 1991). One reason given for this is that girls who menstruate at an early age usually establish an ovulatory cycle at an earlier age and have a higher cumulative exposure to oestrogen. This exposure to oestrogen is believed to be a major determinant of breast cancer risk.

Protection from breast feeding

Recent evidence suggests that breast feeding can protect against the development of breast cancer in young women. In a case control study in the UK, 755 pairs of women were interviewed; one woman in each pair having been diagnosed with breast cancer before the age of 36. The risk of breast cancer fell as the duration of breast feeding increased and also with the number of babies who were breast fed. The benefits of breast feeding continued up until 3 months, but after this period of time there seemed to be no additional benefit from breast feeding.

Age of the menopause

Women who have an early menopause are less at risk of developing breast cancer compared to women who have a later menopause.

Endometrial cancer

Endometrial cancer or uterine cancer as it is sometimes called, occurs most frequently in women aged 55 to 69. It rarely affects women before the menopause and is a fairly uncommon form of cancer. Overnutrition leading to obesity is a major factor in the aetiology of this cancer and the risk increases proportionately as body weight also increases (Doll and Peto ,1981).

Endometrial cancer develops when there is an excessive level of oestrogen in the body and after the menopause the only naturally occurring oestrogens produced are from the adrenal hormones in adipose tissue. At this age therefore, oestrogen levels are directly proportional to the degree of obesity present. As with breast cancer, android obesity – that is obesity concentrated around the upper abdomen and chest – has been shown to be more significantly associated with endometrial cancer than other forms of obesity. Helping women to reduce their weight, if they are obese, is therefore very worthwhile, particularly for those who are susceptible to obesity in the upper part of their body.

Do vitamin supplements offer any protection against cancer?

While there is increasing evidence that the antioxidant vitamins and the trace element selenium have an important role in preventing cancer, there is no evidence to show that women will necessarily benefit from taking these vitamins in addition to a healthy diet. If patients follow the WHO guidelines and consume five portions of fruit and vegetables daily, they should be getting more than adequate amounts of these vitamins and, at the same time, may be consuming other protective factors present in fruit and vegetables which have not yet been formerly identified.

It should be remembered that vitamin A and selenium can be toxic if taken as a supplement in large amounts.

Summary

Diet plays a very significant role in the development of many cancers and the potential for prevention is great. Patients need to be educated about foods that offer protection as well as those that appear to be more harmful. At present a healthy balanced diet is all that is called for and there is no evidence that the general public could benefit from taking vitamin supplements.

Key points – dietary advice

- Include 5 portions of fruit and vegetables in your diet each day
- Avoid having too much saturated fat intake
- Drink alochol in moderation
- Try to maintain a sensible body weight.

Key points – breast cancer

- A low intake of vitamin A may lead to an increased risk of breast cancer
- Being overweight is a risk factor for post-menopausal women – particularly if the weight is concentrated in the upper part of the body
- Breast feeding for 3 months can protect young women against breast cancer.

References

Austoker, J. (1994) Diet and cancer. *British Medical Journal*, **308**, 1610–1614

Dawson, D. (1990) *Women's Cancers The Treatment Options. Everything You Need to Know.* Judy Piatkus Ltd

Doll, R. and Peto, R. (1981) *The Causes of Cancer.* Oxford: Oxford University Press.

Henderson, B. E. and Bernstein, L. (1991) The international variation in breast cancer rates: an epidemiological assessment. *Breast Cancer Research and Treatment*, **18**, 11–17

Hunter, D. J., Manson, J. E., Colditz, G. A. *et al.* (1993) A prospective study of the intake of vitamins C, E, and A and the risk of breast cancer. *New England Journal of Medicine*, **329**, 234–240

Macmillan Breast Cancer Campaign (1994) *Breast Cancer. How to Help Yourself.* London: Macmillan Fund

Rose, D. P., Boyar, A. P. and Wynder, E. (1986) International comparisons of mortality rates for cancer of the breast, ovary, prostate, and colon and per capita food consumption. *Cancer*, **58**, 2363–2371

Schapira, D. V., Clark, R. A., Wolff, P. A. *et al.* (1994) Visceral obesity and breast cancer risk. *Cancer*, **74**, 632–639

United Kingdom National Care Control Study Group (1993) Breast feeding and risk of breast cancer in young women. *British Medical Journal*, **307**, 17–20

Willett, W. (1989) The search for the causes of breast and colon cancer. *Nature*, **338**, 389–394

Willett, W. C., Stampfer, M. J., Colditz, G. A. *et al.* (1990) Relation of meat, fat, and fibre intake to the risk of colon cancer in a prospective study among women. *New England Journal Medicine*, **323**, 1664–1671

Further reading

Tominaga, S. and Kuroishi, T. (1995) Epidemiology of breast cancer in Japan. *Cancer Letters*, **90**, 75–79

Willett, W. C., Stampfer, M. J., Colditz, G. A. *et al.* (1987) Dietary fat and the risk of breast cancer. *New England Journal of Medicine*, **316**, 22–28

World Cancer Research Fund *Think Before you Drink: Alcohol, Cancer and Other Risks.* 11–12 Buckingham Gate, London SW1E 6LB

Chapter 7

Irritable bowel syndrome

Introduction

Irritable bowel syndrome (IBS) is a common disorder which takes up much consultation time in the surgery for nurses, doctors and dietitians. Recent surveys show that it affects about 20% of the general population with more women being affected than men. While it can be experienced by people of all ages women in their 30s and 40s seem to be the group that are most likely to go to their doctor with IBS symptoms.

Contrary to popular medical opinion, patients with IBS are not 'complainers' and many of them put up with their symptoms for months if not years before seeking medical help. In a recent published survey only one-third of patients with IBS symptoms had sought medical advice in the 2 years prior to the survey (Jones and Lydeard, 1992). So why is this? Certainly patients are more likely to seek help if they have a sympathetic GP or feel that their symptoms, such as rectal bleeding, are suggestive of a more serious organic disease. Patients with milder, less worrying symptoms, however, are often put off from returning to the surgery if they have not responded to treatments prescribed in the past from their doctor and feel that there is nothing more that can be done.

Today, alternative therapies such as a change in diet or psychotherapy, are recognized as being valuable in the treatment of IBS and this chapter describes these treatments as well as the pharmacological treatments that are available for patients. Dietary treatment focuses on how high fibre diets can be used and when exclusion diets are appropriate. The last section looks at the role of *Candida albicans* in causing IBS symptoms and describes how dietary advice can help to overcome this.

The diagnosis and symptoms of IBS

Until recently, IBS was only diagnosed after all other possible organic diseases had been ruled out. This involved lengthy, intrusive and often expensive investigations for patients which often caused them considerable anxiety. Today most general practitioners are able to diagnose IBS at the practice without having to refer patients to the local hospital. This is done by looking at their symptoms and measuring them against a standard set of symptoms, often called the Manning criteria.

Here are the symptoms or criteria which make up the irritable bowel syndrome:

- Abdominal pain
- An altered bowel habit
- Relief of pain on defaecation
- Abdominal distension.

The commonest symptom among sufferers is abdominal pain (Maxton, Morris and Whorwell, 1989; Heaton et al., 1992) and this is usually present in the lower abdomen, often occurring in the right or left iliac fossa.

The pain, possibly related to abnormal ileal and jejunal motility, is usually mild to moderate and is recurrent. If there is a prolonged and severe attack the patient may be admitted to hospital where she is usually diagnosed as having 'non-specific abdominal pain' and sent home. Abdominal pain is a very common symptom in the general population and a recent survey found that a significant proportion is believed to be due to IBS. When 1620 people were questioned at random, 25% reported having had more than six episodes of abdominal pain in the preceding year and, in the same sample, 22% also reported other symptoms of IBS. The authors suggested therefore that much of the abdominal pain which is seen in the general population is due to IBS (Jones and Lydeard, 1992).

In addition to colonic symptoms, many people with IBS experience additional symptoms which are now recognized to be part of the general syndrome. These include lethargy, headaches, nausea, dyspepsia, sweating or flushing, mild depression and a feeling of general apathy. To many people these can become as frustrating as some of their bowel symptoms (Table 7.1).

When working with patients who have IBS, it is useful to observe that certain symptoms often occur together. For instance, patients with abdominal pain frequently experience constipation as well and, if dietary treatment is to be offered, taking time to record which group of symptoms a patient is suffering can help to identify which dietary treatment is going to work best.

Table 7.1   Symptoms of IBS in 100 patients

Symptom	Number of patients with the symptom	Symptoms ranked the worst
Abdominal pain	100	30
Abdominal distension	100	6
Abnormal bowel habit	100	20
Contant lethargy	96	14
Backache	75	6
Early satiety	73	1
Excess wind	66	8
Nausea	62	6
Headache	61	2
Urinary problems	56	2
Dyspepsia	51	1
Other symptoms*	20	4

From Maxton, Morris and Whorwell (1989) *British Medical Journal* by kind permission
*These included bad breath, thigh pain, dizzy spells, generalized aches and rectal dissatisfaction.

Here are two groups of symptoms which can sometimes be recognized in patients:

Group 1: abdominal distension, excessive wind, and sometimes but not always loose bowel movements.

Group 2: abdominal pain, sometimes accompanied by constipation.

These two groups will be referred to in Section 5: Dietary treatment.

The causes of irritable bowel syndrome

IBS is a complex heterogeneous disorder and not surprisingly several factors are thought to be involved in its development. For instance, IBS may develop in one patient because there is too much stress in their life, in another because their diet is not suiting them; and in another because of the long-term effects of a particular drug. The recognition that IBS can be caused by many different factors means that, as health professionals, we need to be ready to respond by offering different treatments.

A psychological cause

There is a considerable amount of evidence to support a psychological cause in some patients (Creed, 1994). Psychiatric assessments of patients with IBS have found that large numbers of them score highly for symptoms such as anxiety and depression and in a recent study carried out at St Marks hospital, London, which specializes in disorders of the colon and rectum, many women with IBS admitted to having severe emotional conflicts in their lives (Brook, 1991).

Treatment of IBS aimed at relieving psychological stress can be very effective with good long-term results and in the USA, where psychological factors are more widely recognized as playing a part in IBS, many gastroenterologists provide psychosocial support for their patients. Here in the UK, psychological treatment for IBS varies, including informal group sessions, individual psychotherapy counselling and simple relaxation exercises taught by a physiotherapist. All have been evaluated and have been found to offer lasting relief to a significant number of patients.

A dietary cause

The benefits of using diet therapy to correct the symptoms of IBS is now accepted by the majority of doctors and nurses in the UK. However, it is difficult to say how much an inappropriate diet in the first place is actually responsible for causing the symptoms of IBS. Certainly our diet has changed quite dramatically over the past century: it now includes many refined foods with a high fat and sugar content and it is inevitable that many people will find this difficult to adapt to. In addition to this, many new chemicals have been introduced into our food chain, almost overnight in evolutionary terms, and in the future scientists may discover that this also has an effect on gut function.

Diet is now recognized as playing a significant role in the development of bowel cancer and it should therefore not come as a surprise to us to find that diet can affect the short-term health of the intestinal tract as well. The mechanism is still unclear but the exclusion of certain foods which are difficult for the body to digest and absorb can give very good results. This will be discussed further in the section on dietary treatment.

The pharmacological treatment of IBS

While this chapter is mainly concerned with the dietary treatment of IBS it is useful to describe the main drugs which are prescribed for this condition. These come under five main headings: antidepressants, tranquillizers, antispasmodics or muscle relaxants, bulking agents and peppermint oils (Table 7.2).

Table 7.2   Commonly prescribed drug treatments for IBS

Type	Chemical name	Proprietary name
Antidepressants	Tricyclic antidepressants	Amitriptyline, etc.
Tranquillizers	Benodiazepines	Temazepam, etc.
A combined tranquillizer and antidepressant	Fluphenazine and nortriptyline	Motival
Antispasmodics	Mebeverine hydrochloride, dicyclomine hydrochloride, Hyoscine butylbromide	Colofac Merbentyl Buscopan
Bulking agents	Ispaghula husk	Fybogel Isogel
	Methyl cellulose	Regulan Celevac
Peppermint oil		Colpermin Mintec

Bulking agents and antispasmodic drugs are the most frequently prescribed preparations and have been shown, when given with advice about a high fibre diet, to help about two-thirds of patients. Pharmacological preparations however frequently have draw backs, for example:

- The financial cost to the surgery and patient.
- Unwanted side effects.
- The masking of the real cause of IBS, e.g. psychological or dietary.
- Poor long-term success.

Most patients, when given the choice, prefer to manage their symptoms without taking drugs and this is why psychological support or dietary management of IBS is preferable in most cases. Certain preparations may be useful for treating individual symptoms, i.e. a bulking agent may be used in the short term for constipation, or peppermint oil may be prescribed initially to give relief while a patient starts diet therapy. However, for the long-term relief of *all* the symptoms that occur in the irritable bowel syndrome there is no convincing research to say that any of the drugs currently being used is more successful than a placebo (Klein, 1988).

The dietary treatment of IBS

High fibre diets

High fibre diets have been very popular over the past 20 years and have been prescribed frequently by gastroenterologists and GPs for the treatment of IBS. For some patients this treatment has been very successful, but there is now clinical evidence to show that this type of diet does not suit everyone and for some, a high fibre diet can actually make symptoms worse. It is therefore important that when patients are being given advice it is first established which symptoms they have, as this will help to determine whether or not they will benefit from a high fibre diet.

Here are some guidelines:

Symptoms which may benefit from a high fibre diet:

- hard stools
- constipation
- abdominal pain.

A high fibre diet can help to improve the consistency of hard stools and increase stool frequency in patients who are constipated. It can also help to relieve abdominal pain.

Symptoms which are *unlikely* to benefit from a high fibre diet and may get worse:

- loose stools
- frequent stools
- excessive wind.

What type of fibre should be recommended?

Recommendations for a high fibre diet have changed over the past 5 years. Firstly, the use of processed bran is no longer recommended as it interferes with the absorption of certain minerals in the diet and many patients with IBS actually experience a deterioration in their symptoms when they take bran (Francis and Whorwell, 1994). Secondly, it is increasingly being recognized that some patients with IBS cannot tolerate wholewheat products such as wholemeal bread, Weetabix, Shredded Wheat, branflakes and wholewheat pasta, as these products contain a high concentration of wheat fibre, similar to that found in processed bran. Therefore, patients suffering predominantly with abdominal pain and constipation should be encouraged to follow a diet which includes a wide variety of high fibre foods from other sources, such as oats, brown rice, sweetcorn, potatoes, pulses, large quantities of green and root vegetables, and fresh fruit. They should be advised to experiment with wholewheat products – trying them occasionally until they are sure that they can tolerate them.

Cereal fibre is certainly effective at improving stool consistency but this does not mean that it has to come from wheat products. Fibre from other cereals such as brown rice and oat-based cereals can be just as effective.

Sugar

Many patients with abdominal pain and constipation do not tolerate large amounts of sugar in their diet and a bad attack may come after a celebration or party in which they have eaten a number of foods which are high in sugar. If a patient has followed a high fibre diet for 6 weeks and is still complaining of abdominal pain she should be advised to avoid the major sources of sugar in the diet including cakes, biscuits, chocolates, sweets, fizzy drinks, ice cream, fruit yoghurts sweetened with sugar and sugar added to drinks. This dietary advice can also be very helpful for any patient suffering from dyspepsia or indigestion in the upper part of the digestive tract. I have come across several patients who have not needed to take their antacid preparation after following a sugar-free diet for 3–4 weeks.

Food intolerance and IBS

Food intolerance is now recognized to be a significant cause of IBS in many patients (Jones et al., 1982; Nandra et al., 1989). The link between IBS and food intolerance has been pioneered by many gastroenterologists but particularly by Dr Hunter and his team at Addenbrookes Hospital, Cambridge. They have found that between 40 and 60% of patients with IBS can obtain relief of their symptoms by following an Exclusion diet and then reintroducing foods to find out which are the ones causing the problems. They have found that the fewer the foods allowed on the Exclusion diet, the greater the number of patients who respond, demonstrating that some patients can have some unusual food intolerances (Parker et al., 1995).

Table 7.3   Good sources of dietary fibre (fibre content/100g)

Vegetables	*Cereals*
● Baked potatoes 2.5	● Sweetcorn 5.7
● Cabbage 2.5	● Brown rice 5.5
● Carrots 3.0	● Muesli 7.4
● Broccoli 3.6	● Oat meal 7.0
● Beetroot 3.1	● Wholemeal bread 8.5
● Leeks 3.9	
Nuts	*Pulses*
● Almonds 14.3	● Peas (frozen) 12.0
● Brazils 10.3	● Baked beans 7.3
● Peanuts 8.1	● Lentils (cooked) 11.7
● Walnuts 5.2	● Red kidney beans 25.0
Dried fruits	*Fruit*
● Dates 8.7	● Bananas 3.4
	● Blackberries 7.3
	● Stewed prunes 8.1

NB. Patients with IBS should be aiming for between 25 and 30 g of fibre in their diet each day.

Which patients should be referred to a dietitian to try an Exclusion diet?
It has already been acknowledged that IBS is a complex condition with more than one cause and many treatments which can help. It is therefore important that health professionals are careful to try to identify which patients are most likely to benefit from an Exclusion diet before referring them. This can be done by looking at a patient's symptoms. The list of symptoms which are

Table 7.4   Symptoms most likely to respond to an Exclusion diet

● Diarrhoea
● Abdominal bloating
● Excessive wind
● Abdominal pain

Patients who require an exclusion diet will usually have all or most of these symptoms.

most likely to respond to an Exclusion diet are set out in Table 7.4, with the most important at the top.

Foods which commonly cause problems

Cereal and dairy products are the most common foods which cause IBS symptoms, however coffee, onions, eggs, citrus fruits and chocolate are also common offenders. Unfortunately, many people who embark on an exclusion diet find that they are intolerant to more than one food and this can mean that their normal dietary intake is changed significantly. If they are having to exclude major food items in their diet such as bread, wheat-based cereals, milk and dairy products their diet is likely to become deficient in certain nutrients and they will probably require a nutritional supplement in the long term.

The practicalities of an Exclusion diet

Any patient whom you think may be suffering from a food intolerance and who is keen to identify which food or foods may be upsetting them should be referred to a dietitian. Arranging a suitable exclusion diet is a skilled job and requires time and nutritional expertise. Someone who is experienced in this field can be an invaluable asset to the primary care team. Patients often require support while they are on the exclusion diet and certainly need help during the reintroduction of food items. They will need information on how to adapt their diet when all the foods have been tested and on alternative foods to eat and cook. They will also benefit from having their new diet assessed, to check that it is nutritionally adequate and they may need advice about nutritional supplements.

The extensive use of convenience foods in our diets today makes it difficult for many patients to follow an Exclusion diet and not all patients have the determination or ability to stick to it; about 25% will fall by the way side, including some who feel they cannot afford it.

Tests for food intolerance

There is currently no simple test to measure whether a patient has a food intolerance. Tests for IgE allergy are usually negative and radioallergosorbent (RAST) and skin prick tests can give misleading results (Parker *et al.*, 1995). Some private laboratories use the cytotoxic test, which involves studying a fresh sample of the patient's blood and examining the appearance and motility of live neutrophils when they are exposed to food antigens. If the cells rupture or there is a reduction of movement by the cells, this is used to indicate the presence of a reaction to a food.

Testing for an intolerance to wheat

In the specific case of an abnormal reaction to wheat- and gluten-containing cereals, jejunal biopsies have traditionally been used to diagnose coeliac disease. There is no evidence as yet, however, to show that IBS patients with a wheat intolerance have an abnormal jejunal biopsy. In the future patients may be screened for the antigliadin antibody which is present in serum; whether this will be sensitive enough to detect all cases of a wheat intolerance, however, is still unknown.

Testing for an intolerance to lactose in milk

An intolerance to lactose, present in milk and dairy products, can produce symptoms of abdominal bloating, wind and diarrhoea. Gastroenterologists use the hydrogen breath test to diagnose this intolerance as when a patient is unable to digest and absorb lactose large amounts of hydrogen are produced and this is used to confirm the diagnosis.

Candida albicans

Candida albicans is thought to be responsible, by some practitioners, for some of the chronic bowel symptoms that patients present with and as there is an increasing number of self-help books being published on this, I thought that the subject deserved a mention.

Candida albicans is a yeast which colonizes the intestinal tract shortly after birth and under normal conditions it is kept in check by other intestinal bacteria. However, without these checks it is an opportunist and, if allowed to multiply, is capable of invading large sections of the gastrointestinal tract, producing unwanted toxins which can make a patient feel unwell. Patients who are most at risk from an intestinal *Candida* or bacterial overgrowth include:

- Those who have a malfunctioning immune system, such as ME patients.
- Patients who have recently undergone aggressive anti-cancer treatment as this can disturb the natural gut flora.
- Patients who have been prescribed a long course of steroids.
- Patients who have been prescribed frequent courses of antibiotics.

Excessive colonization by *Candida albicans* and other unwanted bacteria in the gut can lead to abdominal pain, abdominal bloating and often an alternating cycle of constipation and diarrhoea. Patients may also complain of other symptoms, including vaginitis, an itchy skin, fatigue, apathy, mouth ulcers, aching muscles, headaches, mood swings and sore throats (Davies and Stewart, 1987). The presence of these symptoms, together with a change in bowel habit, in most cases, is indicative of an overgrowth of *Candida* or another pathological yeast in the intestinal tract. At present, however, testing for the presence of this yeast is difficult; some specialist clinics now carry out gut fermentation tests, but these are not widely available.

Treatment

The idea that an overgrowth of *Candida* in the intestinal tract can cause certain symptoms, has originated largely from practitioners of alternative medicine and it should therefore not come as a surprise to learn that many popular treatments for the eradication of *Candida* are alternative in nature. Orthodox treatment usually involves the prescription of an antifungal drug such as nystatin or amphotericin for a limited period, however, many patients find that natural treatments, including an adaptation of their diet, are the most successful at providing long-term relief (Jacobs, 1994).

Dietary advice for patients who have symptoms of a *Candida* infection

Patients should be encouraged to follow a sugar-free, high fibre diet as described in the section called High fibre diets on p. 107. In addition to this, those with a severe *Candida* problem may find that they have to restrict the amount of fruit they eat to one fruit a day, as a high intake of fructose, the natural sugar found in fruit, can encourage further *Candida* growth. Most patients with a suspected *Candida* overgrowth find that they cannot tolerate alcohol very well and if possible they should avoid it altogether. If this is out of the question, they should try to avoid beer, lager and wine and keep to spirits mixed with a low calorie soft drink as these drinks seem to cause the least problems.

Many patients suffering from a *Candida* infection will have a compromised immune system and they should be advised to take a multivitamin supplement as well. If after a month of following the diet the patient feels no better they should be referred to a dietitian or practitioner specializing in the treatment of *Candida* for further advice, where a more specific diet may be tried.

Garlic

Several clinical studies have demonstrated that garlic has natural antifungal properties (Ghannoum, 1988). The active components of garlic is a sulphur-containing compound known as allicin: it is present in fresh garlic but is unfortunately only found in very small amounts or not at all in commercial preparations. Patients wishing to try it should use fresh garlic and should crush it raw into dishes before serving. Alternatively, patients can try a product called Allicin Complex which is a commercial preparation containing a number of natural antifungal agents.

Probiotics

Probiotics are cultures of 'beneficial' bacteria sold in capsules which are supposed to colonize the large intestine and help to re-establish a healthy gut flora. Unfortunately, there have been no scientific trials carried out on these products to assess whether they are of any help to patients with *Candida* infections and so it is impossible to recommend them at present.

Summary

Irritable bowel syndrome affects a significant proportion of the population, particularly women. Most patients have more than one symptom when they are diagnosed and the most common symptom is abdominal pain. Some patients respond very well to counselling aimed at correcting a psychological illness, while others respond very well to diet therapy. In order to give a patient the most appropriate dietary advice it is important to look carefully at his or her symptoms first, as these will dictate which diet is the most suitable. Patients whose immune systems have at some stage been damaged by disease or drug therapies, may find that they suffer from an overgrowth of *Candida* or other pathogenic yeasts in their bowel. This can lead to many symptoms and may require antifungal therapy as well as a high fibre, sugar-free diet.

Key points – dietary fibre and IBS

- A high fibre diet is beneficial in patients whose symptoms are predominantly constipation and abdominal pain

- The diet should include fibre from pulses, vegetables, fruit, sweetcorn, potatoes, brown rice and oats

- Patients should be advised to introduce wheat fibre carefully into their diet as this could make their symptoms worse

- Many patients will find the exclusion of sugary foods helps to relieve abdominal pain.

> ## Key points – food intolerance and IBS
>
> - By excluding certain foods 50% of patients with IBS can experience an improvement in their symptoms
> - Patients with diarrhoea, abdominal bloating and excessive wind are the patients most likely to benefit from an exclusion diet
> - All patients who wish to try an exclusion diet should be referred to a dietitian.

Case studies

Case study 1: a patient with constipation and abdominal pain

Situation: Isobel had noticed that her bowel habit had become rather sluggish over the past 6 months but did not think any more about this until she started getting a pain in her lower abdomen about once a week, which seemed to get worse the week before her period. She eventually decided to make an appointment to see her doctor and after being reassured that it was nothing serious she was referred to the dietitian for dietary advice.

Diet: her diet was generally good except at the weekends, when her recent decision to take things easy led to her living on sandwiches, pot noodles, frozen pizzas and packets of biscuits.

Advice: Isobel was advised to make some general changes to her diet at the weekend, including having one cooked meal a day with some fresh vegetables, using brown bread and wholewheat pasta and stocking the house with plenty of fresh fruit so that the biscuits became less of a temptation! Isobel followed this advice for over a month and returned to say how much better she felt and that her abdominal pain had disappeared.

Case study 2: a patient with chronic diarrhoea

Situation: Allison had been suffering from very loose bowel movements since she was 6 years old and she was now 14. Her mother had tried many things and had eventually put it down to stress as it seemed to be worse when she was at school. However, when her GP suggested she saw a dietitian to assess her diet she and Alison were quite happy to do this.

Diet: Alison had a very ordinary diet with no particular fads and there were no foods that she seemed to be eating excessively that might cause the diarrhoea.

Advice: Alison was given an exclusion diet to follow for 10 days. During this time she had no bouts of diarrhoea and was greatly encouraged by this. When she came to introduce the foods back into her diet she found that corn products including cornflour and sweetcorn were causing most of her problems but that onions also had a mild diarrhoetic affect as well. Alison was given advice about the necessary foods to avoid and warned about certain processed foods that could contain cornstarch.

Recommended menus for IBS sufferers experiencing abdominal pain and constipation

(*Please note*: These menus are not suitable for women and men who have a food intolerance.)

The menus below include a wide variety of cereal products, fresh fruit and vegetables which are all high in fibre. Foods which are high in sugar have been deliberately left out as these can cause some patients to experience abdominal pain. In addition to this, products containing a lot of wheat fibre such as Weetabix and wholemeal bread have also been left out as these can exacerbate symptoms in some patients (see Section 5. High fibre diets). Having said this, patients should certainly be encouraged to try these foods at some stage, while being aware that they may not suit them.

Day 1

Breakfast
Porridge
Lunch
1–2 soft grain or white rolls with ham and salad, apple
Evening meal
Chicken and mushroom casserole
Brown rice and broccoli
Natural yoghurt with chopped peach or nectarine and 5 ml honey

Day 2

Breakfast
Cornflakes and a banana
Lunch
Jacket potato with baked beans and a little grated cheese, fruit yoghurt

Evening meal
Grilled fish, new potatoes, peas and carrots
An orange and a handful of almonds

Day 3

Breakfast
Muesli
Lunch
Cottage cheese salad with nuts and raisins
Scone and a pear
Evening meal
Spaghetti bolognaise (try wholewheat pasta one week)
Courgettes
Apple chopped up with natural yoghurt and 5 ml honey

Day 4

Breakfast
Poached egg with soft grain bread toasted
Lunch
Peanut butter sandwich with soft grain bread, carrot and celery sticks
Fruit yoghurt
Evening meal
Lentil curry, brown rice and spinach
Fruit salad

Day 5

Breakfast
Porridge
Lunch
Egg and cress sandwich – try granary or wholemeal bread one week
Banana and handful of hazelnuts
Evening meal
Shepherd's pie using finely chopped vegetables and brown lentils instead of mince, baked beans and cabbage
Stewed apple and a little fresh cream

Day 6

Breakfast
$^1/_2$ grapefruit

Cornflakes
Lunch
Cheese salad, apple and packet of crisps
Evening meal
Pork chop
Jacket potato, ratatouille, sweetcorn
Grapes

Day 7 (Sunday)

Breakfast
Muesli
Lunch
Roast meat or vegetarian choice
Potatoes cooked any way, 2 vegetables
Baked apple with sugar-free custard or fruit salad
Evening meal
Cream cheese and cucumber sandwiches
Toasted teacake

References

Brook, A. (1991) Bowel distress and emotional conflict. *Journal of the Royal Society of Medicine*, **84**, 39–42

Creed, F. (1994) Psychological treatment is essential for some. *British Medical Journal*, **309**, 1647–1648

Davies, S. and Stewart, A. (1987) *Nutritional Medicine. The Drug-Free Guide to Better Family Health*. London: Pan Books

Francis, C. Y. and Whorwell, P. J. (1994) Bran and irritable bowel syndrome: time for reappraisal. *Lancet*, ii, 39–40

Ghannoum, M. A. (1988) Studies on the anticandidal mode of action of *Allium sativum* (garlic). *Journal of General Microbiology*, **134**, 2917–2924

Heaton, K. W., O'Donnell, L. J., Braddon, F. E. *et al.* (1992) Symptoms of irritable bowel syndrome in a British urban community: consulters and non-consulters. *Gastroenterology*, **102**, 1962–1967

Jacobs, G. (1994) *Candida albicans: Yeast and Your Health*. Macdonald Optima

Jones, A. V., Shorthourne, M., McLaughlan, P. *et al.* (1982) Food intolerance: a major factor in the pathogenesis of irritable bowel syndrome. *Lancet*, ii, 1115–1117

Jones, R. and Lydeard, S. (1992) Irritable bowel syndrome in the general population. *British Medical Journal*, **304**, 87–90

Klein, K. (1988) Controlled treatment trials in the irritable bowel syndrome: a critique. *Gastroenterology*, **95**, 232–241

Maxton, D. G., Morris, J. A., Whorwell, J. A. (1989) Ranking of symptoms by patients with the irritable bowel syndrome. *British Medical Journal*, **299**, 1138

Nandra, R., James, R., Smith, H. *et al.* (1989) Food intolerance and the irritable bowel syndrome. *Gut*, **30**, 1099–1104

Parker, T. J., Naylor, S. J., Riodan, A. M. *et al.* (1995) Management of patients with food intolerance in irritable bowel syndrome: the development and use of an exclusion diet. *Journal of Human Nutrition and Dietetics*, **8**, 159–166

Further reading

Trickett S. (1990) *Irritable Bowel Syndrome and Diverticulosis: a Self Help Plan*. London: Thorsons

Workman, E., Hunter, J. and Jones, V. A. (1984) *The Allergy Diet: How to Overcome your Food Intolerance*. London: Martin Dunitz Ltd

Chapter 8
Preconception and nutrition

Introduction

The importance of preconceptional nutrition was first recognized during the Dutch famine of 1944–1945. Infant mortality and morbidity figures which were collected around this period revealed striking differences between infants who had been conceived before the famine, during times of plenty, and those who had been conceived during it. What was particularly interesting was the difference between infants who were *born* during the famine compared with infants who were *conceived* during the famine. Infants who were born during the latter half of the famine but conceived before food shortages began were on average 200–240 g lighter than the previous generation; however no developmental or congenital abnormalities were seen. In contrast to this, infants conceived during the famine had much higher rates of low birthweight, perinatal mortality and a high incidence of congenital malformations.

This historical tragedy served to highlight the fact that an inadequate supply of nutrients around the time of conception is actually more harmful, in terms of infant mortality and morbidity, than an inadequate supply during the latter stages of pregnancy.

This chapter starts by looking at the physiology of fetal development in the first trimester and describes how diet at this stage can affect the health of the baby at birth. There is then a section on practical dietary advice, including the importance of folic acid at the beginning of pregnancy and special dietary advice for women who have been taking the contraceptive pill and women who have insulin dependent diabetes. Finally, there is a practical section which focuses on how to get the message across and including which women to target and what opportunities there are in the community for giving advice.

The physiology of early fetal growth and development

Today the importance of a well balanced diet before and around conception would, I believe, be more readily adopted by women if they were aware of the intense rate of development that takes place within them immediately after conception. During the first 8 weeks (the embryonic period), there is rapid cell duplication with 80% of cell doublings believed to take place before the end of the first trimester. After only 4 weeks a head, body, arm and leg buds are present and a heart can be seen beating. By 6 weeks the embryo has fingers, toes and a liver which can synthesize blood cells. By 8 weeks most, if not all, of the structures and organs are present and ossification has begun in most of the bones. Local stimuli at this time may result in the embryo squinting, opening his mouth or attempting to close his fingers.

During this period, fetal development depends entirely on the endometrium for its nutrient supply because the placenta is not yet formed. Nutrients are laid down in the endometrium during an earlier part of the menstrual cycle – before conception takes place – and then the growing embryo absorbs and digests these nutrients directly. At around 8 weeks the placenta is formed and is able to take over. This dependence upon the endometrium for nutrition at the beginning of life outlines how important it is for a woman to be well nourished before she conceives.

The effect of diet in the first trimester on birth outcome

Traditionally, the effect of a woman's diet on perinatal mortality and birth dimensions has been evaluated by measuring a woman's food intake during the second and third trimesters. This, however, has produced inconclusive results and, except in communities where the quality of the diet is generally poor, the nutritional intake of women during the second and third trimester is difficult to link with birth outcome (Doyle et al., 1992). However, when food intake is measured during the first trimester, there is a positive link between what a mother eats and the health of her offspring. In 1990, Wendy Doyle analysed the diets of more than 500 pregnant women during the first trimester of their pregnancy. At the end of pregnancy the weight, length and head circumference of all the infants were recorded and compared against their mother's nutritional intake. The results showed a clear picture: in infants with birthweights below 3270 g, birth dimensions were clearly associated with a mother's food consumption, i.e. as food intake went up, so too did the birth dimensions. In particular, birthweight and the other dimensions measured, were related to a mother's intake of magnesium, iron and the B vitamins (Doyle et al., 1990).

Further evidence for the role of nutrition came from mothers who produced infants with a very low birthweight, i.e. <2500 g: these mothers were found to have diets which were very low in essential nutritents. Table 8.1 shows a comparison between the diets of mothers who had infants of an optimum weight and those who had infants with a very low birthweight.

It is very important that infants achieve their optimum birthweight, head circumference and body length, as the medical profession has learnt that babies born weighing between 3500 g and 4000 g have fewer congenital malformations and a low perinatal mortality rate. In contrast, babies born

Table 8.1   The mean daily nutrient intakes of 193 London mothers during the first trimester of pregnancy

Nutrient	Mothers of babies < 2500 g (n=28)	Mothers of babies 3500–4500 g (n=165)
Minerals (mg)		
Magnesium	209.00	283.00
Iron	9.35	12.89
Phosphorus	1039.00	1316.00
Zinc	8.16	10.17
Sodium	2026.00	2688.00
Potassium	2493.00	2993.00
Calcium	761.00	953.00
Vitamins (mg)		
Thiamin (B₁)	0.96	1.21
Niacin (B₃)	12.30	16.10
Pantothenic acid (B₅)	3.67	4.41
Riboflavin (B₂)	1.48	1.96
Folic acid (μg)	161.00	201.00
Pyridoxine (B₆)	1.16	1.50
Protein (g)	62.80	74.50
Energy kCal	1642.00	1974.00
kJ	6870.00	8259.00
Fibre (g)	13.50	19.20

(Reproduced from Doyle et al. (1990) *Journal of Nutritional Medicine*, PO Box 25, Abingdon, Oxford, with kind permission)

weighing less than 2500 g have a much greater risk of congenital and neurological malformations and a significantly higher perinatal mortality rate.

In conclusion, a good nutritional intake around the time of conception and during the first trimester, can make a difference to the health of an infant at birth. Every attempt should therefore be made to make sure that women are following a healthy diet at this stage in their pregnancy.

Practical dietary advice

Giving nutritional advice is essentially about recommending foods which are rich in nutrients – particularly the minerals and the B vitamins – and checking that women are having adequate quantities. The following section gives a list of foods which are rich in minerals and B vitamins and a sample menu to see how they can be incorporated.

Foods rich in minerals

Foods which are rich in minerals (iron, magnesium and zinc) include red meat, oily fish, shell fish, pulses and nuts. Women should be eating two to three portions of these foods every day.

Foods rich in B vitamins

Foods which are rich in B vitamins include wholemeal bread, wholewheat chappattis, brown rice, wholewheat pasta, any breakfast cereals, bananas and nuts. Three portions of these foods should be eaten each day. Below is an example:

Sample menu

Breakfast	Weetabix or cornflakes with a banana
Lunch	Tinned salmon sandwiches using granary bread
	Apple and yoghurt
Afternoon	Packet of dried fruit and nuts
Evening	Lentil curry with cabbage and brown rice
	Ice cream and fruit salad
Supper	Milky coffee and digestive biscuit

The above menu illustrates an ideal intake with lentils, fish and nuts providing plenty of minerals and breakfast cereals, granary bread, brown rice, nuts and a banana providing plenty of B vitamins. It is important to realize that this is an ideal, however, and when advising women you may have to be prepared to compromise and be less ambitious in expecting great dietary changes. Below is an example of a very poor diet and how it can be changed into an adequate one.

	Poor diet	*Adequate diet*
Breakfast	Cup of tea	Bowl of cornflakes
Lunch	1 white roll	2 slices Mighty White bread
	tinned soup and packet crisps	with sardines or tuna fish
Afternoon	Chocolate and biscuits	Packet peanuts
Evening	58 g beef burger and chips	113 g beef burger, chips
meal	Yoghurt	and baked beans
		Yoghurt
Supper	Coke and packet of crisps	Glass of milk and packet of crisps

Going through someone's diet in detail can be time consuming and if there is a dietitian in the practice she could be asked for some help. If one is not available, however, asking just a few simple questions and making a few simple suggestions could make quite a difference.

General guidelines to bear in mind when adapting someone's diet

1 First, include some breakfast. (By increasing a persons intake from two meals to three their intake may be increased by a third.) Cereals are the best choice as they are usually supplemented with vitamins and minerals and require milk.

2 The type of bread a person has can make quite a difference to their nutritional intake: if they are not keen on wholemeal or granary breads suggest a high fibre white bread.

3 Packet and tinned soups are poor sources of nutrition. It is better for women to substitute these for some protein, for example in a sandwich.

4 In the afternoon, nuts or fresh fruit are a more nutritious snack than chocolate or biscuits.

5 Many people do not like buying and cooking whole joints or cuts of meat for various reasons. If this is so, it is better to check that adequate portions of processed meat are being eaten than to insist on chops, etc.

6 Baked beans and sweetcorn are popular with many people and should be encouraged as they are an excellent way of increasing the mineral content of a meal.

7 Finally, where food intake is generally of a poor quality, it is wise to recommend a small snack at the end of the day (unless obesity is a problem).

Folic acid and neural tube defects

Since the 1920s it has been recognized that certain deficiencies around the time of conception can lead to disorders of the central nervous system. Iodine deficiency, for example, can result in cretinism and a lack of folate can cause neural tube defects.

In 1991, the Medical Research Council (MRC) published the results of a large study on folic acid supplementation. Nearly 2000 women, at high risk of having a baby with a neural tube defect took part and the results were unequivocal: taking folic acid prevented neural tube defects (Wald *et al.*, 1991).

Today, the Department of Health recommends that all women planning to become pregnant should incrase their folate intakes by eating more folate rich foods *and* by taking 400 μg of folic acid each day.

Table 8.2   Foods rich in folates

Food	Total folic acid (μg)
Spring greens	110
Spinach	140
Canned sweetcorn	32
Dahl	30
Frozen peas	78
Okra	100
Cauliflower	49
Endive	330
Broccoli	110
Brussels sprouts	87
Cabbage Savoy	35
Baked beans	29
Weetabix	50
Muesli	48
Wholemeal bread	39

Prevention

Not every pregnancy is planned, however, and there is a strong case for encouraging *all* women of child bearing age to eat a folate rich diet especially as 95% of all neural tube defects occur as first pregnancies (Czeizel and Dudas, 1992).

The reference nutrient intake (RNI) for folate during pregnancy is 300 μg. Table 8.2 shows some of the foods that are rich in folates and should be included in the diet.

Unfortunately, the message seems to be taking a long time to reach many women. A survey carried out in 1994 of 400 pregnant women found only 2% had modified their diet prior to conception and only 3% had taken folate tablets: *two-thirds* were unaware of the government's recommendations (Clark and Fisk, 1994). Hopefully the public campaign conducted by the Society for Neural Tube Defects has done much to change this.

Giving dietary advice to special groups

Nutritional advice for women coming off the Pill

Some research has demonstrated that over a period of time the contraceptive pill can affect certain blood levels of vitamins and minerals including vitamin A, copper, zinc, vitamin B_6 and folate (Davies and Stewart, 1987). It is therefore important, particularly in the case of folate, that women delay conception for 2–3 months after coming off the Pill. They should be advised to use some other contraceptive during this time and advised to eat a good diet – particularly with respect to their folate intake.

Women with insulin dependent diabetes

A diabetic pregnancy has been described as a high risk state for both mother and fetus (Vaughan, 1994) because many of the usual complications of pregnancy can occur more frequently. These include complications such as infection, hydramnios, pre-eclampsia and placental insufficiency. In addition to this there may be complications associated with the diabetic condition as well. Congenital abnormalities, intrauterine death, macrosomia of the fetus and an increased perinatal mortality are all more common in infants of diabetic mothers. The risk of these complications, however, can be minimized if good metabolic control can be achieved around the time of conception and early on in pregnancy.

Preconceptual and pregnancy care is taken very seriously in diabetic centres where a multidisciplinary team approach is usually used. Once a woman has had her pregnancy confirmed she is usually asked to carry out regular blood glucose measurements at home so that she can try to keep her glucose levels normal throughout the day and be able to monitor the increasing need for insulin that she will have as her pregnancy progresses. Most clinics like women to keep their blood levels between 4 and 8 mmol/l and as more and more diabetic women are able to achieve this, many diabetic centres are now reporting perinatal mortality rates which are similar to those in the non-diabetic population (Vaughan, 1994).

Dietary management of insulin dependent diabetes is important and all patients should ideally see a dietitian at least once during their pregnancy. The diet should be made up of regular meals with a high carbohydrate content, about 200–250 g a day, and unrefined carbohydrates such as wholemeal bread, potatoes, brown rice and wholegrain cereals are recommended as they help to stabilize blood glucose levels and provide the body with a good supply of B vitamins and magnesium.

Healthy carbohydrate foods to include in the diet
Breakfast cereals
Bread
Scones and teacakes
Jacket potatoes
Brown rice
Pasta
Fruit
Fruit yoghurts
Dried fruit and nut mixtures.

Women should be encouraged to have regular meals or snacks throughout the day and should also have something at night before they go to bed as this will prevent them experiencing any hypoglycaemia at night or ketosis in the morning.

On days when women are involved in more physical activity they should be advised about the need to consume extra carbohydrate. When blood glucose levels are being very tightly controlled, as they are in pregnancy, any small change in activity level may bring about a significant fall in blood glucose level and women should be aware of the risk of hypoglycaemia. This of course need not be a problem if they are prepared and always carry a carbohydrate snack around with them.

Getting the message across

How to target women who are at risk of a poor pregnancy outcome

Certain women are much more at risk of a poor pregnancy outcome than others, for obstetric and social reasons. The following section discusses four groups of women who are at risk and it is hoped that in the future a greater proportion of public health resources may be spent on targeting these groups. The four groups include:

- Women from lower socioeconomic groups.
- Women who have already had one low birthweight infant.
- Women who are underweight before they conceive.
- Women who have short intervals between their pregnancies.

Women from low socioeconomic groups
Studies have shown that the rate of perinatal mortality is greatest among families from a lower socioeconomic background (Table 8.3).

There are obviously many reasons for this trend, but current research suggests that differences in diet may be one factor to explain the greater perinatal mortality which seems to exist among lower social groups. One study which supports this theory noticed that intakes of protein, many minerals and B vitamins gradually decreased in pregnant women as their social class became lower (Wynn *et al.*, 1994). This is particularly worrying when studies have shown how important these nutrients are for fetal growth.

Unfortunately, many young women have very poor diets with much of their energy coming from crisps, chocolate, white bread, sweetened tea and biscuits. A poor education, lack of money, inadequate accommodation and an acceptance by society that there is little wrong with these foods, are all

Table 8.3   Perinatal mortality (OPCS, 1994)

Social class	Rate/1000 births
I	6.7
II	7.4
IIINM	8.1
IIIM	8.1
IV	9.6
V	10.7

Reproduced from Office for National Statistics

factors which have allowed these eating patterns to continue. Education by the primary health care team must be a priority with low income families and especially young women, if the perinatal mortality figures are ever to change.

Women who already have an obstetric history of low birthweight

Women who already have one low birthweight baby are particularly at risk of having another: one study found that one in three women goes on to have another baby of low birthweight. This is compared to the national average in which the risk is 1 in every 14 births (OPCS, 1990). These women have experienced at first hand the extra anxieties involved in caring for a low birthweight baby and it is hoped therefore that they may be more open to advice.

Education can be shared by health visitors and midwives who will skilfully need to avoid suggesting that a mother is in any way to blame for her first baby's low weight, while at the same time suggesting that she may like to take an active role in trying to influence the weight of her second baby. Health visitors calling in to check on the first baby's development should be aware that another might be being planned in the future and could take this opportunity to explain to the mother about the importance of a good diet. Good communication with the midwife can ensure that this message is reinforced again during antenatal care.

Women who are underweight at the start of their pregnancy

Women who are underweight before starting their pregnancy are more at risk of carrying a growth retarded or low birthweight infant. In one study underweight women who ovulated spontaneously were three times as likely to have infants who were small for gestational age compared to the control group (van der Spuy et al., 1988). Pre-pregnancy weight is therefore important in determining a healthy birth outcome. A BMI of 20 is the very lowest weight at which a woman should try to conceive while a BMI of 24 is argued to be the optimum weight for pregnancy (see Chapter 10: Infertility). Women trying to conceive when their BMI is less than 20 should be advised to gain some weight before trying again.

Giving advice to this group may be quite difficult because many women enjoy being slim and while they may have prepared themselves for the inevitable weight gain *during* pregnancy, the idea of gaining weight before hand may seem unacceptable. Women with anorexia nervosa are a group particularly at risk from having an infant of low birthweight. After a period of infertility they may enter a transitional period called the penumbra when fertility returns despite their body weight still being very low. Unfortunately, although they may be able to conceive it is unlikely that they will have the nutritional reserves for adequate fetal growth. In this situation, it is best that a patient and her partner should be aware of the dangers of conceiving until her weight is greater.

Women who have short intervals between their pregnancies
Birth spacing is a topic worth discussing with mothers as experience tells us that women who have short intervals between their pregnancies are more likely to have smaller infants and to deliver prematurely (Rawlings, Rawlings and Read, 1995). Adequate time between births is also important so that a mother has time to regain her strength; stores of nutrients, especially iron and folate can become depleted during pregnancy and time is needed to replenish these. If there is an inadequate period between one birth and the next her nutrient status may become depleted and she may feel tired and exhausted during the next pregnancy.

The benefits of a good diet during the interpregnancy interval have recently been demonstrated in the USA where the Women Infant and Child (WIC) programme provides many postpartum women with healthy food items such as milk, cheese, cereals, eggs and fruit juices. Experience has shown that women receiving this food go on to have second infants with higher birthweights and birth lengths and the risk of them having an infant weighing less than 2500 g is significantly reduced. The mothers themselves also benefit by having higher haemoglobin levels at the start of their second pregnancy and suffering less from obesity (Caan *et al.*, 1987).

So how long should a woman wait before having another baby? The answer is we do not know. One study, which looked at nearly 2000 women found that the interval may differ according to race. For black women an interpregnancy interval of less than 9 months was associated with a greater prevalence of low birthweight and prematurity; while only intervals of less than 3 months were associated with a poor outcome among white women (Rawlings, Rawlings and Read, 1995). Until more research is carried out common sense must prevail.

Opportunities for giving preconceptual advice

Opportunities for giving preconceptual advice rarely occur naturally. Most women wait until they are pregnant before attending the surgery and in the few months prior to this it is usually a personal time for a couple when medical help is rarely sought. While to many it may seem like an invasion of privacy to ask questions about conception when a patient has merely called in for a routine medical check, there *are* other times when the subject of preconceptional health could easily be introduced.

Family planning clinics

In theory, any discussion about contraception or infertility treatment should include a brief introduction about the importance of diet in the event of conception. While it may not be information that the patient uses immediately, it may be stored and remembered later when the time is appropriate. Sensitive questioning about a person's current relationship may prompt her to discuss hopes for children in the future and this provides an opportunity to remind her of the importance of diet when that time comes. Every woman deserves a simple education on the importance of diet at the beginning of her pregnancy and, although many may forget to act upon the advice before conceiving, if they start during the first few weeks the reward, 9 months later, could be very significant.

Slimming groups

Slimming groups run by members of the primary health care team are also good opportunities for introducing the issue of diet and pregnancy – albeit as a side issue. Many women attending these groups are in the middle of having families and will be interested in finding out what sort of diets they should be following. Some women may actually be attending the group because their doctor has advised them to lose weight before embarking on another pregnancy.

Important: if a woman is actively trying to conceive *and* wants to reduce her weight at the same time, she should be advised to avoid foods high in sugar and fat such as biscuits, cakes, pastries, chocolate, crisps and chips. She should *not* cut down on cereals, bread, potatoes, meat, vegetables, dairy products and fruit.

High schools

As with many health education programmes the need to start at a young age is increasingly being recognized. Britain has one of the highest incidences of teenage pregnancies in Europe and, although the emphasis for this group is always going to be prevention, teenagers should recognize the importance of their diet if they do become pregnant. This subject could be dealt with in health education or on child care courses.

Summary

The experience of the Dutch famine and recent discoveries in embryology have highlighted the importance of periconceptional nutrition and a balanced diet is now recognized to be essential for ensuring adequate fetal growth and the achievement of optimum birth dimensions. Dietary advice should be given to all women but especially to those who are most at risk. These include:

- Women in low incomes
- Women who are underweight
- Those who have recently given birth
- Those who have an obstetric history of low birthweight infants.

Opportunities for giving advice exist at family planning clinics, slimming groups and higher education establishments.

Key points – dietary advice

Women should:

- Eat two to three portions of meat, oily fish, shell fish, pulses or nuts daily
- Eat three to four portions of wholemeal bread, wholewheat chappatis, brown rice, bananas, breakfast cereals, whole wheat pasta or nuts daily
- Take 400 μg of folic acid before and for 12 weeks during their pregnancy
- Eat a green vegetable daily
- Delay conception 2–3 months after taking the Pill
- Gain weight if their BMI is < 20
- Allow an adequate interval between pregnancies
- Monitor their blood glucose levels if they are diabetic.

Case study

Situation: Annie was referred for dietary advice when she spoke to her GP about trying for another baby. Her previous baby had weighed less than

3000 g at birth, despite being born at full term and so her GP thought it might be a good idea to check that her diet was adequate.

Diet: her diet consisted of a daily cheese sandwich made with white bread, usually an apple in the afternoon and in the evening a variety of traditional cooked meals based around potatoes with minced beef, sausages, fish fingers or turkey steaks. The only vegetables she would eat were carrots, courgettes and tinned tomatoes. At bed time she would often have an ice cream from the freezer.

Advice: Annie was told that her diet probably had sufficient energy in it, as well as protein, but was low in magnesium and the B vitamins, including folic acid. She was advised to change to wholemeal or brown bread and to eat at least three slices a day. She was also advised to eat some dried fruit and nuts every day as a snack and to have a bowl of cereal at bedtime as well as, or instead of an ice cream.

Menus

The following menus include a variety of foods which are good sources of protein, minerals and the B vitamins – all essential nutrients for fetal growth. The meals have been designed to be fairly inexpensive and reasonably quick to prepare.

Day 1

Breakfast
2 Weetabix with milk
Lunch
Cheese sandwich with 2–3 slices of bread
1 banana
Evening meal
Chicken casserole with onions and mushrooms
Potatoes and cabbage
Fruit yoghurt and biscuit

Day 2

Breakfast
1 bowl of muesli with milk
Lunch
Tuna fish sandwich with 2–3 slices of bread
1 orange

Evening meal
Gammon steak with leeks, sweetcorn and new potatoes
Ice cream and stewed fruit

Day 3

Breakfast
1 large bowl of cornflakes and a banana
Lunch
Chicken salad with a medium to large jacket potato
Evening meal
Baked beans on toast, 2–3 slices
Piece of cake and glass of milk

Day 4

Breakfast
1 large bowl of Rice Krispies and an apple
Lunch
Egg sandwich with 2–3 slices of bread
Yoghurt and biscuit
Evening meal
Spaghetti bolognaise with broccoli
Banana and glass of milk

Day 5

Breakfast
2 Weetabix with milk
Lunch
Grilled bacon, poached egg and 2–3 slices of bread
1 apple
Evening meal
Lentil curry or vegetable chilli using kidney beans
Brown rice
Yoghurt and an orange

Day 6

Breakfast
1 bowl porridge made with milk
Lunch
Cottage cheese sandwich

Scone or teacake
Evening meal
Grilled herring or cod steak or fish fingers
Parsley or cheese sauce, potatoes, peas and carrots
Fresh fruit salad

Day 7 (Sunday)

Breakfast
Large bowl cornflakes with milk and banana
Lunch
Roast meat, roast or boiled potatos, and two vegetables – including a green vegetable
Any dessert
Evening meal
Egg sandwich
Piece of cake

References

Caan, B., Horgen, D., Margen, S. *et al.* (1987) Benefits associated with WIC supplemental feeding during the interpregnancy interval. *American Journal of Clinical Nutrition*, **45**, 29–41

Clark, N. A. and Fisk, N. M. (1994) Minimal compliance with the Department of Health recommendation for routine folate prophylaxis to prevent fetal neural tube defects. *British Journal of Obstetrics and Gynaecology*, **101**, 709–710

Czeizel, A. E. and Dudas, I. (1992) Prevention of the first occurrence of neural tube defects by periconceptional vitamin supplementation. *New England Journal of Medicine*, **327**, 1832–1835

Davies, S. and Stewart, A. (1987) *Nutritional Medicine. The drug-free Guide to Better Family Health*. London: Pan Books

Doyle, W., Crawford, M. A., Wynn, A. H. A. *et al.* (1990) The association between maternal diet and birth dimensions. *Journal of Nutritional Medicine*, **1**, 9–17

Doyle, W., Wynn, A. H. A., Crawford, M. A. *et al.* (1992) Nutrition counselling and supplementation in the second and third trimesters of pregnancy, a study in a London population. *Journal of Nutritional Medicine*, **3**, 249–256

Office of National Statistics (1996) Mortality Statistics, Childhood, infant and perinatal, 1993 and 1994, England and Wales. Series DH3, no. 27, p. 245

Rawlings, J. S., Rawlings, V. B. and Read, J. A. (1995) Prevalence of low birth weight and preterm delivery in relation to the interval between pregnancies among white and black women. *New England Journal of Medicine*, **332**, 69–74

van der Spuy, Z. M., Steer, P. J., McCusker, M. *et al.* (1988) Outcome of pregnancy in underweight women after spontaneous and induced ovulation. *British Medical Journal*, **296**, 962–965

Vaughan, N. J. A. (1994) Diabetes in pregnancy. *Current Obstetrics and Gynaecology*, **4**, 155–159

Wald, N., Sneddon, J., Densem, J. *et al.* (1991) Prevention of neural tube defects: results of the Medical Research Council Vitamin Study. *Lancet*, ii, 131–137

Wynn, S. W., Wynn, A. H. A., Doyle, W. *et al.* (1994) The association of maternal social class with maternal diet and the dimensions of babies in a population of London women. *Nutrition and Health*, **9**, 303–315

Further reading

Advice on preparing for pregnancy – an excellent leaflet produced by the Mother and Baby Clinic, 189 Well Street, Hackney, London E9 6QU

Cunningham, F. G., Macdonald, P. C., Leveno, K. J. *et al.* (1993) *Williams Obstetrics*, 19th edn. London: Prentice Hall International

Thomas, B. (ed.) (1994) Pregnancy. In: *Manual of Dietetic Practice*, 2nd edn, pp. 255–256. Oxford: Blackwell Scientific Publications

Chapter 9

Infertility and body weight

Introduction

Infertility is usually investigated when a woman has been having difficulty conceiving for about 2 years and while 80% of couples manage to conceive within the first year of trying, between 10 and 15% of couples are known to experience problems with their fertility. This, according to health statistics is a higher incidence compared to three decades ago and can partly be explained by changing social trends including the delay of childbirth, the use of the intrauterine device (IUD) and the increased incidence of salpingitis which has accompanied the greater sexual freedom among women in recent years.

Being underweight can also greatly reduce a woman's chances of conceiving and the object of this chapter is to discuss how nutritional advice can help women who are underweight increase their fertility. The advice in this chapter is meant to be supplementary to any medical treatment.

The influence of body weight on fertility

Women who are underweight are much more likely to experience problems with their fertility than women who are of an average weight or women who are overweight (Wynn and Wynn, 1990). They are also recognized as being more at risk of having more preterm pregnancies and low birthweight infants (van der Spuy et al., 1988). Research into the subject has found, not suprisingly, that fertility is normally at an optimum level when a woman's BMI is between 23 and 24. This is an average weight to height ratio which is recommended for good general health normally. If a woman's body weight begins to fall below this level it appears that her fertility also starts to decrease. The relationship between fertility and body weight seems to be continuous below this point, i.e. the lower it drops below 23 the more likely it is that a woman will be infertile and at a BMI of between 18 and 20 it is estimated that only 50% of women are able to conceive (Wynn and Wynn, 1990). Below a BMI of 18 most women are starting to experience problems with amenorrhoea.

Inducing ovulation in underweight women

Women who fail to ovulate regularly each month are often treated with gonadotrophins which artificially induce ovulation. While this can be very effective in helping women conceive, their use is now thought to be unwise in women who are underweight as it carries too great a risk for the fetus (van der Spuy et al., 1988). The problem with inducing ovulation in underweight women is that, although their infertility can be corrected, their nutritional status is often poor and as a consequence they are not able to sustain a healthy pregnancy. Experience has shown that underweight women, especially those who have had ovulation induced, frequently deliver preterm babies who are of a low birthweight. In one study, women with a BMI below 19.1, who required ovulation to be induced, were recorded as having a fivefold increase in the risk of having a baby with a birthweight below the 10th centile (van der Spuy et al., 1988).

Because of the many medical problems associated with infants of a low birthweight many gynaecologists are now unhappy about inducing ovulation in women who are underweight and may insist that women achieve their normal body weight before prescribing the appropriate drugs.

Infertility in women who have been following a weight-reducing diet

Women who lose a significant amount of weight after following a weight-reducing diet may experience a temporary disruption to their menstrual cycle and as a result find that conception is difficult for a few months afterwards. This is most likely to happen if the weight loss has been sudden or the diet has not been of a nutritionally high standard and should not normally occur in women who follow a moderate balanced diet. If this situation does occur women should be advised to stop their diet and encouraged to eat normal quantitites of healthy food for 2–3 months *before* trying to conceive again.

Giving nutritional advice to women who are infertile

Nutritional advice is useful for all women with fertility problems but especially for women who are underweight. For these women the advice should consist of two messages, with the second being the most important:

- Increase your body weight
- Eat large quantities of nutrient rich foods.

Some women are unable to increase their body weight significantly despite eating very large quantities of food and although this is unfortunate they should not be too concerned. While the body's reproductive system is certainly sensitive to body weight as it decreases, research shows that it is *more* sensitive to the composition of the diet being consumed and therefore if women are eating large quantities of nutrient rich foods it is possible for them to override the negative effects of their weight. This fact was highlighted in a study of 513 pregnant mothers living in Hackney where two very thin mothers with a BMI of 16–17 conceived and unexpectedly produced babies who weighed more than 3 kg. This was a very good outcome for such thin women and could only be explained by the fact that their diets were exceptionally good (Wynn and Wynn, 1990).

Practical dietary advice

The following advice should help women with fertility problems to gain weight and ovulate naturally each month. While following this advice they should weigh themselves once a week and after one month should return to the surgery to discuss their progress.

Recommendations

1 Try to eat three meals a day and one snack – a regular intake of food is important.
2 Do not use low fat products such as skimmed milks and low fat margarines.
3 Fill up on healthy snacks such as sandwiches, cheese and savoury biscuits, yoghurts, fruit, and cereals rather than chocolate, sweet biscuits, cakes and crisps.
4 Nuts are a particularly handy snack to carry around and are high in calories and minerals.
5 Not all fats are unhealthy and the use of vegetable oils can be recom-

mended for frying meat, fish, potatoes or making salad dressings. This will increase the number of calories in a meal significantly.

Summary

Women who are significantly underweight find it much more difficult to conceive and therefore any woman who is underweight and thinking about starting a family should be given dietary advice first. This will not only increase a woman's chances of conception but also improve her chances of having a healthy baby of an optimum weight at the end of her pregnancy.

Key points

- Women are generally most fertile when their weight is at a healthy average (BMI between 23–24)

- Fertility is reduced in women who are underweight and at a BMI of 18–20 only 50% of women are fertile

- Drug therapy used to induce ovulation is not recommended in women who are underweight as it carries too great a risk to fetal development

- Women who have been following a very strict weight reduction programme may experience a temporary disruption to their menstrual cycle

- Nutritional advice to women who are underweight is important not only in aiding conception but also in helping a healthy pregnancy outcome.

Case study

Situation: Jenny had been trying for a baby for 8 months when she came to see her doctor for some advice. Her general health was good but her weight was low at 46 kg (7st 3lb) and when her height was measured her BMI was only 18. Her doctor explained that this was probably why she had not conceived and recommended that she discuss her diet with the dietitian.

Diet: Jenny's diet consisted largely of high calorie carbohydrate snacks such as doughnuts, crisps, biscuits and lots of chocolate as she thought this would help her to put on some weight.

Advice: it was explained to Jenny that by eating a more balanced diet she would be more likely to conceive and also to provide the right nutrients for the growth and development of her baby. So she was recommended to have a bowl of cereal if she felt hungry, rather than some chocolate; a sandwich with some protein in it at lunch time and a cooked meal in the evening including a green vegetable. Jenny was also advised to have a milky drink sometime during the day.

References

van der Spuy, Z. M., Steer, P. J., McCusker, M. *et al.* (1988) Outcome of pregnancy in underweight women after spontaneous and induced ovulation. *British Medical Journal*, **296**, 962–965

Wynn, A. and Wynn, M. (1990) The need for nutritional assessment in the treatment of the infertile patient. *Journal of Nutritional Medicine*, **1**, 315–324

Chapter 10
Pregnancy

Introduction

This chapter is designed to give midwives and practice nurses up-to-date information about the nutritional needs of women during the second and third trimesters of their pregnancy. (The nutritional needs of women during the first trimester has already been discussed in Chapter 8). While it is the midwife who normally takes responsibility for this stage of a woman's life, it is also useful for practice nurses to be aware of the nutritional needs of pregnant women and so this chapter has been written with both student midwives and practice nurses in mind.

The chapter focuses on the following areas:

- The nutritional requirements for women during the last two trimesters of pregnancy.
- Weight gain during pregnancy.
- The management of women with gestational diabetes.
- The need for iron supplements.
- The importance of a good intake of magnesium.
- Advice for special groups, such as adolescents and vegetarians.

(A food checklist is available at the end of the chapter which can be used to assess the adequacy of a woman's diet in the clinic.)

Background physiology

By the end of the first trimester most of the fetal organs are present and the placenta is functioning. Growth, rather than organ development is now the dominant process and the demand for nutrients to sustain this growth begins to increase. The main physiological processes which demand a specific supply of nutrients are:

- The production of blood cells in the fetal liver and bone marrow which requires large amounts of iron.
- The ossification of fetal bones in the last 3 months which requires considerable amounts of calcium.
- The growth of all fetal tissues which requires protein and energy.
- Brain and neurological development, which takes place primarily in the last trimester and which requires a supply of essential fatty acids.

While there is a steady increase in fetal length throughout gestation, body weight, however, does not show a linear pattern of growth. In the first trimester fetal weight gain is very small and can hardly be measured; then after the 12th week there is a gradual increase followed by a tremendous spurt of growth in the last 2 months, when fetal weight is almost doubled. During these last 2 months extra energy is required to support this growth and many women find that they are naturally inclined to eat more at this time.

Dietary requirements in pregnancy

(NB. This is a large section for those particularly interested in the role of individual nutrients. For a quick summary of the dietary requirements during pregnancy, refer to the end of this section where the information is summarized in Table 10.2.)

Energy

The energy cost of pregnancy has been estimated to be 70 000kcal (293 MJ) over the 9 months, but most studies have found that women rarely increase their intake by this much. The supply of nutrients for fetal development always takes precedent over a mother's own needs during pregnancy and unless maternal energy intakes and fat stores are severely low, fetal growth will progress normally. It is only women suffering from anorexia nervosa or those who are underweight at the start of their pregnancy *and* who continue to have a poor food intake who are likely to have inadequate energy supplies to support their own, and their babies' requirements during the pregnancy.

While individual appetites can vary throughout pregnancy, most women notice a natural increase in their appetite during the last few weeks and the Department of Health certainly recommends that women increase their energy intake in the last trimester by 200 kcal a day (Department of Health, 1991).

In practice: women do not need to eat a greater quantity of food when they are pregnant except in the *last* trimester when they will normally experience an increase in appetite anyway. Women should have an additional sandwich or bowl of cereal each day, rather than making up the extra 200 kcal with biscuits and chocolate which have very little nutritional value.

Groups at risk: drug addicts and patients suffering from anorexia nervosa may be at risk from an inadequate energy intake and regular contact with these women can help to monitor the situation. Women from ethnic minorities should also have their diets assessed, ideally by a dietitian, as some research has shown that many have inadequate energy and nutrient intakes during their pregnancy. (See Chapter 12 on the needs of ethnic minority groups.)

Protein

The additional requirement for protein in pregnancy is very small – 6 g per day. This means that woman's total protein requirement increases to 51 g per day.

In practice: most adult women already have an adequate protein intake which will easily cover this additional need so no change to the diet is needed.

Groups at risk: women who follow a vegan diet may be the only group who are at risk and they should be encouraged to eat plenty of soya products, pulses and nuts each day so that their protein requirements are being met.

Calcium

There is no recommendation to increase calcium in the diet during pregnancy because the absorption of calcium by the mother's gut increases greatly.

In practice: women should be encouraged to have an adequate intake of dairy products in their diet including 284 ml milk and 30 g of cheese or a yoghurt each day to give them a basic intake of around 550 mg of calcium. The rest of their requirement will usually come from green vegetables, bread and cereals and normal quantities of these foods each day will make their total intake up to 700 mg which is the recommended nutrient intake (RNI) set for calcium (Department of Health, 1991). (When checking a person's calcium intake it should be remembered that compared to brown and white bread, wholemeal bread is a poor source of calcium and if this is being eaten all the time it may be advisable to recommend a slightly higher intake of dairy products, nuts or green vegetables to compensate for this. Wholemeal bread also contains large amounts of phytate which can bind calcium in the gut and prevent it being absorbed.)

Groups at risk: women who are intolerant to dairy products and pregnant adolescents both need specialist advice and should be referred to a dietitian where possible. Those who are intolerant to dairy products should be advised to take a calcium supplement while they are pregnant and this may need to be increased if they plan to breast feed. Adolescents, on the other hand, do not need a supplement but should be encouraged to take extra calcium in the form of milk, cheese, or yoghurt each day. Adolescents should be drinking or consuming 584 ml milk every day during their pregnancy so that they meet their higher RNI of 800 mg calcium per day.

Magnesium

(See an additional section on magnesium, p. 152).

Magnesium plays a very significant role in fetal development in the first trimester but does not seem to be so critical during the second and third trimesters (Doyle *et al.*, 1992). It may, however, have a role to play later on in pregnancy that we are currently unaware of and so women should be encouraged to continue having a good intake of foods rich in magnesium, not least, so that their own health does not suffer.

In practice: women should be encouraged to eat a variety of foods which are good sources of magnesium every day, for example green leafy vegetables, pulses, wholegrain products, dried fruit and nuts.

Groups at risk: women on a low income who are eating a very refined diet.

Iron

Iron is needed in increasing amounts during pregnancy for fetal growth, development of the placenta and the increase in maternal red blood cell production. This demand is met in two ways: first from maternal stores laid down before pregnancy and secondly through the increase in iron absorption which occurs during pregnancy (Table 10.1).

Because of these natural adaptations, a normal healthy diet is all that is required and routine iron supplementation is no longer recommended. Recently there have been concerns expressed about routine iron supplementation to otherwise healthy women and in a recent midwifery publication two trials are sighted in which iron supplementation resulted in an increased incidence of preterm births and low birthweights. The authors suggested that this may have come about because of an increase in the viscosity of maternal blood which, in turn, may have impeded uteroplacental blood flow (Enkin *et al.*, 1995).

Table 10.1 Percentage of non-haem iron absorbed from food during normal pregnancy in 12 healthy subjects

Subject number	Weeks of gestation			After delivery
	12	24	36	
1	3.1	16.1	71.5	36.8
2	3.4	23.3	59.4	–
3	4.3	27.4	72.1	15.3
4	4.7	53.0	83.6	5.2
5	5.0	20.0	38.8	–
6	5.7	44.1	70.5	15.8
7	6.2	37.1	73.9	4.9
8	12.8	52.7	80.9	–
9	14.2	51.3	85.9	19.3
10	14.4	46.4	49.3	13.4
11	14.9	44.2	68.9	4.7
12	16.2	54.4	63.9	–
Geometric mean	7.2	36.3★	66.1★	11.3

★Mean was significantly ($P < 0.001$) higher than preceding value
(Reproduced from Barrett *et al.* (1994) *British Journal of Medicine* by kind permission)

In practice: women should be encouraged to eat a balanced diet with a regular intake of meat or pulses, fish and green vegetables. They should be discouraged from drinking tea or coffee with meals as this reduces iron absorption and should drink fruit juices instead. The following foods are rich in iron and every woman, pregnant or not, should try to include two of these foods in her diet each day: fortified cereals, brown bread, pulses such as baked beans or kidney beans, red meat, sardines, nuts and dried fruit.

Women who may be at risk of developing an iron deficiency
Women who start their pregnancy with poor iron stores and who continue to have a low intake of dietary iron can become anaemic. These are usually women who have not eaten very well for several months, often for economic reasons, but sometimes as a result of depression. Other groups who are also vulnerable are:

- Adolescents
- Those with a poor vegetarian diet
- Women who have conceived very soon after a previous pregnancy.

Detecting genuine aneamia in pregnancy is difficult as haemoglobin levels fall naturally during pregnancy as a result of the expansion in plasma volume, often referred to as hypervolaemia of pregnancy. Instead of assessing haemoglobin levels therefore, the measurement of mean cell volume is a much more accurate reflection of iron deficiency as it is not closely related to haemoglobin concentrations and declines quite rapidly in the presence of an iron deficiency (Enkin *et al.*, 1995).

Women who are found to have a microcytic anaemia are normally given an oral iron supplement to correct the deficiency and at the same time advice should be given about which foods are rich in iron so that the problem does not recur.

Dietary advice for women who develop anaemia

- Avoid drinking tea and coffee with meals.
- Have diluted fruit juice instead.
- Eat wholegrain or fortified cereals and brown or wholemeal bread.
- Vegetarians should try to eat pulses at least three times a week.
- Meat eaters should include some red meat in their diet unless they are eating plenty of pulses.
- Nuts are a good snack to have in between meals.
- A green leafy vegetable should be included with the main meal most days.

B vitamins

Most people in the UK consume adequate amounts of the B vitamins in their diet, and the slight increase which is required during pregnancy is met in all but the very poorest of diets.

In practice: women do not need to make any changes to their diets.

Groups at risk: alcoholics or those eating a very poor, highly refined diet that does not contain any whole grain products or fortified cereals may be at risk. They should be persuaded to have some brown or wholemeal bread and if possible a wholewheat or fortified cereal each day. If any woman is unable to do this they should be given a vitamin B supplement to take throughout their pregnancy.

Folate

(See section on Folate and Neurotube defects in Chapter 8.)

Folate requirements increase significantly during pregnancy because of the increased cell turnover and if there is insufficient folate in the diet in the second two trimesters of pregnancy, a women can develop a deficiency which can lead to megaloblastic anaemia. Today, most women receive a folic acid supplement during the first trimester to avoid neural tube defects in the growing fetus but they should be aware of the importance of continuing to have a good dietary intake of folate throughout the latter part of their pregnancy for the preservation of their own health.

In practice: all women should be encouraged to eat plenty of green leafy vegetables, pulses, and have a fortified or wholegrain breakfast cereal every day.

Groups at risk: women on a low income.

Vitamin C

During pregnancy the demand for vitamin C gradually increases and is greatest in the last trimester. It is therefore recommended that women who are pregnant increase their intake of this vitamin from 30 mg to 50 mg a day.

In practice: most women already have an adequate intake of vitamin C but it is useful to check that some fruit is being eaten especially among women on a low income. Cirtus fruits, melons and strawberries are particularly good sources of vitamin C but potatoes also contain small amounts and are of course a cheaper source of the vitamin.

Groups at risk: women who smoke will have even higher daily requirement for vitamin C and should be encouraged to eat plenty of fruit.

Vitamin A

Additional vitamin A is required throughout pregnancy for growth and maintenance of the fetus and an extra 100 μg is recommended by the Department of Health to meet this demand.

In practice: however, most women in the UK already have plenty of vitamin A in their diet and so there is no need for women to increase their intake of foods which are rich in this vitamin. Very high intakes of vitamin A of more than 3300 μg/day are thought to cause congenital birth defects and as a precautionary measure women are advised *not* to take supplements which contain vitamin A during their pregnancy. The Department of Health has also advised women not to eat animal livers, as recent research has found them to contain extremely high levels of vitamin A; 13 000–40 000 μg/100 g depending on the species (Department of Health, 1991). Livers from organically reared animals however are safe to be eaten and are a good source of iron.

Vitamin D

The action of sunlight on the skin is the single most important supplier of vitamin D for most people rather than any food in the diet. However, foods such as fortified margarine and oily fish do provide an additional small amount and can be important during the winter months when exposure to sunlight is limited.

In practice: there seems no reason why sunlight should not continue to be the main provider of vitamin D during pregnancy and to ensure this happens women should be encouraged to get plenty of fresh air.

Groups at risk: Asian women are at risk of having low vitamin D levels in their blood due to a combination of dietary factors and low exposure to the sun and so they are recommended to take a vitamin D supplement at all times and especially if they are pregnant. Similarly, Scottish women are also recommended to take a vitamin D supplement when they are pregnant as research has shown that their infants are more likely to develop hypocalcaemia, dental enamel defects and hyperparathyroidism if they do not take this supplement (Department of Health, 1991).

Conclusion

Physiological changes during pregnancy are designed to increase the delivery of nutrients to the fetus and in the majority of cases this naturally ensures that the nutritional requirements for growth and development are easily met. However, there are some women, particularly those on a low income, whose diets are low in certain nutrients, especially iron and magnesium and these women are at risk of becoming nutritionally depleted during their pregnancy. To avoid this, women whose diets are generally poor or erratic, should receive some dietary advice.

Weight gain in pregnancy

The amount of weight which is gained during pregnancy can vary greatly, ranging from a loss to a gain of around 23 kg or more. The majority of

Table 10.2   Summary of the dietary requirements during pregnancy

Nutrient	Reference nutrient intakes	In practice	Groups at risk
Energy	1940 kcal + 200 kcal in last trimester	Eat to appetite in last trimester	Some women from ethnic minority groups, those with a history of anorexia nervosa, drug addicts
Protein	51 g (a 6 g increase)	Most diets adequate	Vegans
Calcium	700 mg – no increase	Check that intake of dairy produce is adequate	Adolescents, those intolerant to dairy products
Magnesium	270 mg – no increase	Check intake of green vegetables, nuts, whole grain cereals	Women on a low income
Iron	14.8 mg – no increase	Check intake of cereals, brown bread, red meat	Women who drink tea or coffee with meals
B vitamins	Increase 0.1 mg B_1 (last trimester only) Increase 0.3 mg B_2	Most diets adequate	Those with *very* poor diets, alcoholics – give supplement
Folate	300 μg – increase of 100 μg	Eat a green vegetable daily	Women on a low income
Vitamin C	50 mg – increase of 10 mg	Eat 1–2 fruits daily	Women who smoke
Vitamin A	700 μg – increase of 100 μg	Most diets are adequate, high intakes can be teratogenic	Women should not take vitamin A supplements or eat animal livers
Vitamin D	10 μg – increase of 10 μg	Sunlight will be the main source	Asian and Scottish women. These women should take supplement

*Figures are taken from the Department of Health published in 1991.

women, however, gain around 12.5 kg. Excessive weight gain is not encouraged during pregnancy as it has been associated with the development of gestational diabetes, pre-eclampsia and hypertension, and for this reason most obstetricians and midwives are careful to monitor weight gain during the last two trimesters. What is more contentious, however, is whether women who begin their pregnancy with a body mass greater than 30, should aim for a smaller increase in weight than their normal weight counterparts. An extensive piece of research carried out two decades ago certainly supports this idea, concluding that it reduces the perinatal mortality rate in this group (Naeye, 1979). However, many midwives today are of the opinion that a more relaxed approach should be taken towards weight gain, especially when in some women it is obviously related to oedema.

A balanced, individual approach to giving dietary advice therefore needs to be employed; encouraging women to eat sensibly but at the same time making sure that they do not become too concerned about their weight.

Practical advice for women who are overweight at the start of their pregnancy

Restricting excessive weight gain in the obese patient can be done very safely and simply; advising them to restrict foods which are high in energy but low in essential nutrients such as biscuits, cakes chocolate and crisps. Women should be encouraged to have a more natural diet instead made up of protein foods, cereals, vegetables and fruit. These foods are not high in calories and contain plenty of nutrients needed by the growing fetus.

Dietary advice

- Have three meals a day.
- Eat fruit in between meals when hungry.
- Choose carbohydrate foods which are high in fibre, e.g. wholemeal bread, brown rice, jacket potatoes, etc.
- Avoid high fat and high sugar foods, e.g. chocolates, cakes, biscuits and crisps.
- Do not restrict quantities of milk, meat, fish, potatoes, bread, cereals, fruit, vegetables and nuts in the diet.

This diet should not be seen as a 'reducing diet' but as a healthier diet which will automatically have less calories in it.

Conclusion

Medical and midwifery opinion remains divided about restricting food intake in pregnancy. However, there is no evidence to suggest that encouraging women to follow a healthier diet has any detrimental effect on fetal growth and most women welcome the positive effect it has on controlling any excessive weight gain.

Gestational diabetes

Gestational diabetes mellitus (GDM) is an intolerance to glucose which occurs during pregnancy. It is usually diagnosed in the second or third trimester and is much more common in ethnic minority groups, particularly in women from the Indian subcontinent (Dornhorst *et al.*, 1992).

The adverse outcome most frequently associated with GDM is fetal macrosomia and up to 30% of mothers with an abnormal glucose tolerance test have infants with a birthweight of 4000 g (Enkin *et al.*, 1995). However, measuring a woman's glucose tolerance is not the only way of forecasting fetal macrosomia as other factors such as maternal weight before pregnancy and weight gain during pregnancy are also very useful in predicting this condition. As a result many obstetricians question the value of testing glucose tolerance levels during pregnancy, especially as it can cause unnecessary anxiety among some women.

Testing is also viewed with scepticism by many obstetricians and midwives because research has so far failed to establish that treatment with diet and or insulin actually reduces perinatal deaths. In a review of the literature carried out at the Fetal Centre at Liverpool Maternity Hospital it was found that neither a controlled diet nor insulin therapy appeared to offer any significant advantages to women with GDM or their babies and it was therefore concluded that at present screening of all pregnant women seemed unnecessary (Walkinshaw, 1993). What the review did establish, however, was that there is a clear association between GDM and obesity and therefore it seems sensible to advise that any woman who is obese at the start of her pregnancy should receive a few simple dietary instructions so that she does not experience excessive weight gain during her pregnancy which may exacerbate the situation.

Dietary advice for women with GDM who are overweight

- Cut down on foods containing large amounts of sugar, e.g. cakes, biscuits, sweets, chocolates, puddings, fizzy drinks and ordinary squashes.

- Choose unrefined carbohydrates such as wholemeal bread, brown rice, wholewheat pasta, wholewheat crackers and fresh fruit.
- Eat fruit in between meals.
- Keep foods with a high fat content to a minimum, e.g. crisps, chips, pastries.

(NB. It is important, that women with GDM do not restrict their energy intake significantly, as this may cause them to produce ketones. This could have a detrimental effect on fetal growth and development (Magee, Knopp and Benedetti, 1990).)

Lifestyle advice for women after their pregnancy

After pregnancy, the majority of women find that their glucose levels return to normal. Unfortunately, however, research shows that approximately half of these women will go on to develop an impaired glucose tolerance or non-insulin dependent diabetes within 10 years of their pregnancy (Dornhorst, 1994). Women with GDM should therefore be counselled after their pregnancy so that they are aware that this might happen and understand which symptoms they should look out for. The importance of treating diabetes as early as possible cannot be overstated as an impaired glucose intolerance is a very important risk factor for coronary heart disease in women and the sooner it is treated the greater the chance there is of preventing cardiac and circulatory complications. Various lifestyle changes can help to prevent or delay the development of diabetes in women who have developed GDM during their pregnancy and they should be encouraged to come and discuss these changes after their pregnancy.

Practical advice for women after their pregnancy

1 Try to achieve a sensible weight for your height, e.g. body mass index of around 25.
2 Stop smoking.
3 Take some regular exercise.
4 Have your blood glucose levels checked every 2 years.
5 If you are planning to have another baby have your blood glucose level checked before conceiving.

Magnesium: a mineral of importance

For health professionals who are interested in future developments and research, there is increasing evidence that magnesium may have a greater role in birth outcome than was originally thought. In a study of more than 500 women who were either given 15 mmol magnesium or a placebo daily the authors found that magnesium supplementation was associated with a reduction in the number of preterm deliveries and fewer referrals to the neonatal intensive care unit (Spatling and Spatling, 1988). If supplementation is ever to be considered for clinical practice these results need to be repeated; and the stage in pregnancy when supplementation should begin also established.

At present, however, midwives should check that all pregnant women are including some magnesium rich foods in their diet each day by using the checklist below.

Magnesium checklist
Include two foods from the list each day:

- A wholegrain breakfast cereal – Weetabix, Shredded Wheat, muesli, porridge, branflakes
- Brown, wholemeal or granary bread
- Sweetcorn
- 60 g nuts
- Baked beans or another pulse vegetable
- Brown rice
- 60 g dried fruit.

Giving advice to adolescents who are pregnant

Adolescents who became pregnant have large nutritional requirements: they require a considerable intake of nutrients and energy to meet their own growth and development and an additional intake for their baby's growth and development. This translates into a large intake of food each day. The benefits of eating a large quantity of food is not always an easy message to get across, particularly when many young girls are very conscious of their figures and have often been used to restricting their food intake on a daily basis, to achieve an ideal body weight.

Recommending a healthy diet can also be difficult: many teenagers are not very concerned about eating healthily and strong peer pressures at this age can make it very difficult for girls to be different. Despite these difficulties, however, every attempt should be made to explain the importance of eating well during pregnancy and how it can benefit both her and her baby. It should be pointed out that eating well does not necessarily mean an enormous baby at the end – an important fact for many girls who may be quite apprehensive about giving birth!

The eating pattern of teenagers is frequently oriented towards snacking and typical foods include chips, sandwiches, biscuits, crisps, beef burgers, and sausage rolls. Eating times may be erratic with many going without breakfast or skipping lunch and generally teenage girls tend to have poorer nutritional intakes than boys simply because they do not consume the same quantity of food that boys do. Nutritional advice for this group needs to be simple and unambitious and encouraging girls to suggest ways themselves in which their diets could be healthier, may result in better compliance. Here are some ideas as to how to improve an adolescent's diet.

Practical dietary advice

1 Check that *enough* food is being eaten.
2 Accept that snacking is an important way of eating in this age group and try to find ways of making snacks healthier:
   - suggest eating nuts or chocolate raisins rather than crisps
   - suggest a cereal bar rather than a bar of chocolate
   - suggest fruit or a bowl of any cereal rather than biscuits.
3 Encourage wholemeal or soft grain bread sandwiches rather than white bread and a protein filling rather than salad or jam.
4 Encourage 568 ml milk a day or 284 ml and a yoghurt and/or some cheese each day.
5 Always discourage them from going long periods without food.

Common problems in pregnancy

Coping with nausea

Nausea occurs in at least half of all pregnancies and is considered to be quite normal. Psychological and hormonal changes have both been suggested as possible causes, along with vitamin deficiencies and a change in the metabolism of carbohydrate foods. Nausea usually starts around the 6th to 9th week of pregnancy and has gone by the 16th week, although some women can feel sick throughout their pregnancy.

Nausea is often worse when the stomach is empty and relief is usually achieved by eating something starchy (Table 10.3). Women should be encouraged to eat small high carbohydrate snacks at regular intervals throughout the day and to keep a glass of fruit juice by their bedside which can help with nausea first thing in the morning. Anecdotal evidence from women suggests that aeriated drinks can also be helpful.

Table 10.3   Snacks to relieve nausea

Wholewheat toast and Marmite or jam
Fresh fruit salad
Jacket potato with tuna or baked beans
Cottage cheese and roll
Plain biscuits
Soup and crackers
Scones or teacakes

If symptoms are severe women should try taking a vitamin B complex supplement. In all cases, women should be reassured that nausea is a normal part of being pregnant and that it is unlikely to last for long. If they are finding it difficult to eat very much they should be reassured that regular healthy snacks can be just as nutritious as cooked meals.

Heartburn

This is another common problem in pregnancy which usually occurs in the third trimester. Women can minimize the discomfort by having smaller meals and soon learn to identify specific foods that are causing them problems (Table 10.4).

Occasionally citrus fruits and bananas can also cause heartburn and if, after cutting out the foods below, there is still some discomfort women should be advised to try avoiding these fruits as well.

Alcohol

Avoidance of alcohol at the very beginning of pregnancy is a wise precaution as it is well known that excessive drinking at this stage leads to fetal alcohol syndrome, a condition characterized by mental and physical retardation. After the first trimester, however, the occasional drink is not thought to have any detrimental effect on fetal growth or development (Thomas, 1988).

Table 10.4   Foods which commonly cause problems

Fizzy drinks
Fatty foods – chips, crisps, pastries, fried food
Spicy food

Listeriosis

Materno-fetal listeriosis is a bacterial infection that is thought to result in spontaneous abortions, stillbirths and the delivery of an infected baby. Although it is an uncommon infection in pregnancy, an overall rise in the number of human infections during the 1980s has prompted the Department of Health to issue guidelines to pregnant women on the avoidance of certain foods which are considered to be contaminated by the bacteria.

These are the foods that women are advised to avoid:

- Soft ripened cheese such as brie, camembert and blue veined cheeses
- All types of pate
- Cook chilled meals such as quiches, unless they are thoroughly re-heated
- Ready to eat poultry.

The Department of Health has also recommended that women pay adequate attention to food hygiene and in particular to check the 'use-by' dates on perishable foods.

Summary

Most women have a diet which adequately provides for the growth of their baby in the second and third trimesters. However, some women, including adolescents and those on a low income, frequently have diets which lack some of the essential nutrients and as a result of the significant metabolic demands of pregnancy, these women risk becoming nutritionally depleted by the end of the third term. To prevent this happening, extra support and information should therefore be provided for them about inexpensive nutritious foods that they can buy and the quantities of food that they should be consuming each day.

Key points

- Look out for groups at risk: those on a low income, alcoholics, women from ethnic minority groups and adolescents. Refer these women to a dietitian

- For other women use the checklist at the end of the chapter to assess their diet   (continued opposite)

(continued)

- Women who are overweight at the start of their pregnancy should be given dietary advice to help them avoid excessive weight gain
- Women with gestational diabetes who are overweight should also be given dietary advice.

Checklists

Below are two lists which can be used to quickly assess a woman's diet in the last two trimesters of pregnancy. One is designed for meat eaters the other is for vegetarians. They are simple to use and can check the adequacy of a woman's diet in a few minutes.

Checklist 1 for women who eat meat

A healthy diet should include the following each day:

1 serving of meat or fish
1 serving of cheese or eggs or pulses
2 servings of bread, breakfast cereals, pasta or rice
(preferably wholegrain varieties)
1 serving of potatoes
2 servings of other vegetables (including a green leafy vegetable)
2 portions of fruit or 1 glass of fruit juice
568 ml milk or 1 yoghurt and 30 g hard cheese
Some butter or margarine (fortified with vitamin D)
(Adapted from Thomas, B. (ed.) (1988) *Manual of Dietetic Practice*, Blackwell Science Ltd, by kind permission)

Checklist 2 for women who are vegetarians

A healthy diet should include the following each day:

2 servings of cheese or eggs or pulses or nuts
2 servings of bread, breakfast cereals, pasta or rice (preferably wholegrain varieties)
1 serving of potatoes
2 servings of other vegetables (including a green leafy vegetable)
2 portions of fruit or 1 glass of fruit juice
568 ml milk or 1 yoghurt and 30 g hard cheese
Some butter or margarine (fortified with vitamin D)

Case studies

The following two case studies are examples of the sort of nutritional problems that a midwife or dietitian might come across.

Case study 1: fatigue and constipation

Situation: Helen was referred for dietary advice when she was 20 weeks pregnant as she was complaining of fatigue and constipation and wondered whether her diet was lacking in anything.

Diet: Helen followed a vegetarian diet eating a variety of foods including pulses, nuts, cheese, eggs, green and root vegetables and soya products. She had three meals each day and a sandwich at supper. Despite having white bread she had plenty of fibre in her diet from vegetables and pulses which she ate daily. Her drinks consisted of tea, water and the occasional gin and tonic.

Advice: Helen was congratulated on her good diet and reassured that her symptoms of tiredness and constipation were probably due to the hormonal changes that occur during pregnancy. However, to reassure her it was decided that she should be investigated for iron deficiency by measuring her mean cell volume and serum ferritin levels. (These are more sensitive tests for iron deficiency than measuring blood haemaglobin levels.) In the mean time she was advised to stop drinking tea with or near her meals and recommended to have diluted fruit juice instead. To help relieve her constipation she was advised to try some wholemeal bread, have a citrus fruit or some prunes each day and to drink plenty of water.

Case study 2: advice to a young girl living on a low income

Situation: Andrea was 20 years old and living in a women's refuge when she was referred for dietary advice. Her income was limited and her knowledge of nutrition was poor.

Diet: her nutritional intake consisted largely of white sliced bread, crisps, cup-of-soups and chocolate biscuits. In the evening she usually made herself something on toast except at weekends when she would grill a beefburger, some fish fingers or a chop and would do some frozen vegetables and oven chips to go with it. Her GP had prescribed an iron and folate supplement for her which she was taking.

Advice: Andrea was encouraged to cook a further two meals during the week and to think about sharing the cooking with another woman in the refuge once a week. She was advised to have large helpings of vegetables with these meals. Andrea was also encouraged to increase her intake of dairy foods by having cheese and biscuits for a snack at supper time and by having milky drinks of Ovaltine and hot chocolate throughout the day rather than cups of tea or soup. Cereal bars, fruit and chocolate raisins were recommended as snacks in preference to crisps. Finally, Andrea was persuaded to try some cereal for breakfast instead of having toast, as it was explained to her that this would be of greater nutritional value.

Andrea was seen by the dietitian 2 weeks later and was making a start at changing her diet. She was seen again 2 weeks later and then, with the support of her GP, it was decided that she no longer required the iron and folate supplement.

Low budget healthy menus for pregnant women

The following menus are cheap and simple to prepare and where possible use fresh ingredients rather than convenience food as it is usually cheaper and of higher nutritional value. Wholegrain cereals and bread are obviously preferable but not essential if women are not keen. Cereal is included in most menus as it utilizes milk and is generally a more nutritious option for breakfast compared to toast and marmalade.

Day 1

Breakfast
Breakfast cereal with full fat milk
1 slice of toast with jam or marmalade
Lunch
Cheese on toast (2 slices)
Apple
Evening meal
Shepherd's pie
Baked beans and carrots
Tinned fruit and custard

Day 2

Breakfast
Breakfast cereal with full fat milk
1 slice of toast with Marmite
Lunch
Baked beans on toast (2 slices)
A glass of fruit juice and a wholemeal teacake

Evening meal
Fish fingers (4)
Potatoes, peas and cabbage
Rice pudding

Day 3

Breakfast
Breakfast cereal with full fat milk
1 slice of toast with a boiled egg
Lunch
Corned beef sandwich (2 slices)
Banana
Evening meal
Stir fried vegetables: carrots, onions, sweetcorn, mushrooms, cauliflower and tuna with brown rice
Glass of milk and a digestive biscuit

Day 4

Breakfast
2 slices toast with Marmite
Lunch
Cheese salad with coleslaw
Piece of fruit cake and an apple
Evening meal
2 sausages
Potatoes, peas and carrots
Angel Delight

Day 5

Breakfast
Cereal with full fat milk
1 slice toast with peanut butter
Lunch
Cottage cheese and tomato sandwich
Banana and digestive biscuit
Evening meal
Chicken casserole using thigh portions
Potatoes and cabbage
Tinned or fresh fruit and custard

Day 6

Breakfast
Cereal with full fat milk
Banana
Lunch
Tuna fish and tomato sandwich
Piece of fruit cake
Evening meal
Jacket potato with cheese and baked beans
Fruit yoghurt

Day 7

Breakfast
Scrambled egg on 2 slices of toast
Lunch
Roast meat of any choice or a vegetable curry
Potatoes or rice, 2 vegetables
Sponge pudding and custard
Evening meal
2 toasted crumpets with jam
An apple and a banana

References

Barrett, J. F., Whittaker, P. G., Williams, J. *et al.* (1994) Absorption of nonhaem iron from food during normal pregnancy. *British Medical Journal*, **309**, 79–82

Department of Health (1991) *Dietary Reference Values for Food Energy and Nutrients for the United Kingdom*. Report on Health and Social Subjects 41. London: HMSO

Dornhorst, A. (1994) Review: implications of gestational diabetes for the health of the mother. *British Journal of Obstetrics and Gynaecology*, **101**, 286–290

Dornhorst, A., Patterson, C. M., Nicholls, J. S. D. *et al.* (1992) High prevalence of gestational diabetes in women from ethnic minority groups. *Diabetic Medicine*, **9**, 820–825

Doyle, W., Wynn, A. H. A., Crawford, M. A. *et al.* (1992) Nutritional counselling and supplementation in the second and third trimester of pregnancy, a study in a London population. *Journal of Nutritional Medicine*, **3**, 249–256

Enkin, M., Keirse, M. J. N. C., Renfrew, M. and Neilson, J. (1995) *A Guide to Effective Care in Pregnancy and Childbirth*, 2nd edn. Oxford: Oxford University Press

Magee, M. S., Knopp, R. H. and Benedetti, T. J. (1990) Metabolic effects of 1200 – kcal diet in obese pregnant women with gestational diabetes. *Diabetes*, **39**, 234–239

Naeye, R. L. (1979) Weight gain and the outcome of pregnancy. *American Journal of Obstetrics and Gynecology*, **135**, 3–9

Spatling, L. and Spatling, G. (1988) Magnesium supplementation in pregnancy: a double blind study. *British Journal of Obstetrics and Gynaecology*, **95**, 120–125

Thomas, B. (ed.) (1988) Pregnancy. In: *Manual of Dietetic Practice*. Oxford: Blackwell Scientific Publications

Walkinshaw, S. A. (1993) Diet and insulin vs diet alone for 'gestational diabetes'. In: *Cochrane Database of Systematic Reviews*: review no. 26650. Cochrane Updates on Disk, Oxford: Update Software, 1994, Disk Issue 1.

Chapter 11

Helping low income families choose a healthy diet

Introduction

Ever since the Black Report in 1982, health professionals have realized that people on a low income have much higher mortality rates from most recorded illnesses and are generally much more vulnerable to ill health than people who have an average or above average income. In particular, a low income has come to be associated with an increased incidence of coronary heart disease, cerebrovascular disease and some diet-related cancers; and many people who are employed in the field of health promotion now spend much of their time trying to find ways to respond to this problem.

Poverty can affect general health in many ways, for example people on low incomes are much more likely to live in homes with environmental problems such as damp and heavy pollution from traffic fumes. They may find it difficult to heat their homes adequately, pay for preventive dental and ophthalmic services, buy adequate protective clothing and footwear and of course find extra money for a healthy diet. These are some of the more obvious consequences of having a very limited income but there are also many other, less obvious effects of being poor that can bring about a chronic level of ill health. For example, the stress of being out of work for a long time, or of continually having to deny your children things that other children are able to have, can also lead to ill health.

Unfortunately, many people who suffer from long-term poverty and who see little hope of their situation ever changing often gain relief from smoking or drinking and this of course brings additional health problems. When looking specifically at diet and poverty it is clear that eating a healthy diet is only seriously considered by people when their income is sufficient for them to feel financially secure. In other words, when the basic commodities of life such as a house, car and clothes have become affordable, without too much hardship, people then begin to think about their health and in particular what they can do to ensure good health for the future. If people do not achieve this financial security, they are very unlikely to appreciate the value of spending their scarce resources on their health especially when there are usually no immediate benefits.

For some the reality is black and white: a healthy diet is simply unaffordable. A single mother with two children for example, living in rented accommodation on Income support, will have little extra money to spend on luxuries and any savings she can make on food bills may be important to her for putting towards a much needed new bed or a week's holiday in the summer for her and the children. For her, a healthy diet is a luxury that she feels she cannot afford.

The following chapter looks at what low income families are eating today and takes a look at the cost and availability of a healthy diet. As the elderly are particularly vulnerable to poverty their problems are also discussed. The last section is devoted to a summary of points to remember when giving practical dietary advice.

What do people on a low income eat?

Fruit and vegetables

Figures from the 1991 *National Food Survey* by MAFF, show that the distinguishing trait between the diets of middle income people and those with a low income is the lack of fruit and vegetables in the diets of the latter group. All social classes are still consuming too much fat, but it appears that those on a low income are at an even greater risk of common diseases such as heart disease because they are not consuming sufficient fruit and vegetables. To eat more of these foods is perhaps the most important message that can be conveyed to low income families as they are such a valuable source of antioxidant vitamins, fibre and some minerals.

One reason why families may be reluctant to eat more fruit and vegetables is for a practical reason – they are heavy to carry. One study reported that women found them bulky to carry home (Gibney and Lee, 1993) and this cannot be dismissed as an insignificant factor when many families on a low income have to rely on public transport. To obviate this problem families should be encouraged to shop at local markets where fruit and vegetables are cheapest and do not need to be carried long distances home. Alternatively, in some areas there are mobile delivery vans which sell fresh produce directly to residential areas.

Fat intakes

While the overall fat intake of all social groups is still too high, people in the lower income groups tend to consume more of the wrong sort of fat. Their main intake of fat comes from spreadable fats (which are often not polyunsaturated), biscuits, cakes, pastries, sweets and chocolates (Gibney and Lee, 1991), which is different to other income groups where the main sources of fat are usually dairy produce, meat and spreadable fats. Low income families should therefore be encouraged to use a polyunsaturated margarine on bread and in cooking rather than margarines which contain a high proportion of saturated fat. They should also be given advice about the high fat content of biscuits and pastries.

Sugar intakes

Sugar intakes are higher in low income groups than middle or upper income groups. In a study carried out among a group of unemployed people in Dublin some women were found to be having as much as 190 g of table sugar a day (Gibney and Lee, 1991). Much of this sugar is often used to sweeten hot drinks and it can be a useful first step, when discussing a healthier diet with someone, to see if they can reduce the sugar in their tea or coffee.

The cost and availability of a healthy diet

Cost of a healthy diet

Healthier food choices are frequently more expensive than the foods which we are being recommended to reduce in our diets; and there is genuine evidence to suggest that it is a real lack of money, rather than ignorance, that leads most people to buy an inferior diet. In a study on the subject of poverty and nutrition carried out by the charity NCH Action for Children, people were asked what foods they would buy if they had an extra £10 a week: 60% said that they would buy more fruit, 54% more lean meat and 38% more vegetables. This is unequivocal evidence that people know what they should be doing, but feel unable to do so for financial reasons.

Many people argue that eating a healthy diet is not any more expensive than eating an unhealthy one but, when the facts are looked at, this can easily be disproved. In a study, carried out by a dietitian based at the Royal Free Hospital (Mooney, 1990), the costs of two baskets of food were compared: one containing foods recommended for a healthy diet and the other containing foods not recommended for a healthy diet (see Table 11.1).

Table 11.1   Shopping baskets used for costing (all weights 500 g)

Shopping basket A Recommended foods in a healthy diet	Shopping basket B Foods to be reduced in a healthy diet
Cottage cheese	Cheese spread
Edam cheese	Cheddar cheese
Semi-skimmed milk	Whole milk
Polyunsaturated margarine	Soft margarine
Polyunsaturated vegetable oil	Ordinary vegetable oil
Wholemeal bread	White bread
Weetabix	Cornflakes
Brown rice	White rice
Wholewheat spaghetti	White spaghetti
Wholemeal flour	White flour
Tinned beans, low sugar	Tinned beans, added sugar
Tinned peaches, no added sucrose	Tinned peaches, added sucrose
Low fat burgers	Ordinary burgers
Low fat mince	Ordinary mince
Low fat sausages	Ordinary sausages

(Reproduced from Mooney (1990) *Journal of Human Nutrition and Dietetics* by kind permission of the Publishers, Blackwell Science Ltd, Oxford)

When the prices of food were analysed in nine shops across Hampstead, London basket A was found to cost 18% more than basket B. This is quite an increase if you are someone who is keeping to a tight budget.

The other interesting piece of information that came out of the study was that buying healthier food in the more deprived areas of Hampstead was proportionately more expensive. Although foods were generally cheaper from these shops than foods purchased in shops from the more affluent areas; the *difference* in cost between the healthy basket of food and the less healthy basket was greater than 21%. Proportionately therefore, poorer people wishing to buy healthier foods were having to pay more (Mooney, 1990).

It can therefore be concluded that switching to a healthier diet does involve spending more money and that for those living in deprived areas of suburban developments, the difference between purchasing a healthy basket of food and an unhealthy one may be considerable.

How available are healthy foods?

Not all food stores sell a wide variety of healthy food choices and the above study found that in general supermarkets and shops in the deprived areas of Hampstead were less well stocked with healthy foods. In one large supermarket five out of the 15 healthy choices in basket A were not available. This contrasted with food stores and supermarkets in the more affluent areas where a greater variety of health foods was stocked, catering for individual preferences.

The energy content of a healthy diet

What should also be remembered when advising families on a low income to switch to a healthier diet is that many foods which are recommended are foods which are relatively low in energy; for example fruit and vegetables, low fat milks, low fat cheeses and low fat yoghurts are all fairly low in calories. If a person is to keep their energy intake the same, they will have to buy more of these foods which of course will increase their food bill even more. If a person is overweight this is not such a problem as they are trying to reduce their energy intake anyway, but a mother who has four growing children to feed may feel that spending money on fresh fruit which has a very low energy content, is an expensive way of filling her children up. Biscuits on the other hand are high in energy and therefore a more economical way of meeting her family's energy needs.

Cooking skills

Cooking skills are in short supply across the whole social strata today but people with little money often lack the confidence as well as the facilities to experiment with food and so tend to rely more heavily on convenience foods. Many will not have had much advice from their parents about food preparation and will be afraid that their cooking may turn out to be inedible and wasted as a result. A family with a limited budget cannot afford to waste food and so many see convenience meals as a safer option.

Most women with children are, however, open to the idea of learning basic cooking skills and practical cookery sessions are usually very successful at helping women to change their family's food intake. Several dietitians up and down the country are involved in community projects in which women are invited to cook and taste foods and then discuss their nutritional value;

some are even involved in setting up cooperatives in which healthy food can be purchased at more affordable prices (Department of Health, 1994). Certainly more practical cookery sessions with women and also men who are interested, are needed in the community if the parents and grandparents of the future are to gain some confidence about cooking.

The elderly

Some of the elderly living in England number among Britain's poorest residents and they are perhaps the group most at risk from malnutrition. As well as living on a low income many have physical disabilities and this makes food preparation difficult. In addition to this, many have no transport of their own which means that they either have to struggle on public transport with heavy shopping or have to shop locally where the choice of food may be limited and more expensive.

Social isolation also makes many older people less inclined to bother very much with the preparation of meals and a casual glance at an old person's shopping basket in a supermarket trolley frequently reveals that much of their pension is spent on biscuits, cakes, bread and jam. These are high energy, relatively cheap foods which require little preparation and have a long storage life – a significant consideration for people living on their own when their turnover of food is not very great. However, these foods have very little nutritional value apart from being a good source of energy and with time a person living exclusively on these foods will become ill.

An additional problem for the elderly is that food which is bought in small quantities is always more expensive than larger packs aimed at families. Thus, elderly people living on their own who wish to follow a healthy diet are penalized twice: first they must pay more for the healthier food choices and secondly they must pay more because they are buying small quantities of food.

Encouraging older people to buy adequate amounts of fruit and vegetables, lean meat, fish and dairy products can be difficult, especially when these are perishable items. However, there are ways to overcome some of these problems. For instance it could be suggested that they do their shopping with a friend with whom they could share some of the larger items. Alternatively, most old people have a small freezer section in their fridge and this could be used to stock small amounts of meat or frozen vegetables. Products such as tinned fish, eggs and cheese have a long storage life, and can be bought cheaply in small amounts. These are excellent sources of protein and can quickly be made into a nutritious snack without much effort. Most elderly people are interested in their health and are keen to do anything that will help them stay well; in my experience most welcome some advice about their diet.

How to go about discussing dietary changes with patients on a low income

First, encourage people to have more fruit and vegetables in their diet. This is the most important piece of advice you can give. Explain how it can be protective against heart disease and cancer and suggest that they try buying these products from a market stall where it is usually cheaper.

Ask patients what foods they would like to buy if they had more money available to them. This can be a good way of discussing the sort of healthy foods that they like and may lead them to suggesting possible ways in which they could include some of these foods in their diet, say by replacing one unhealthy food for a healthier one.

Patients are often reluctant to try new foods but are happy to try healthier alternatives of the products they are used to. For example, they may be happy to try tinned fruit in natural juice rather than tinned fruit in syrup or low fat sausages rather than ordinary sausages, if these are the foods they are used to. Simple changes like these could make a significant difference to their diet in the long term.

Try to understand the reasons why people are reluctant to spend extra money on a healthy diet; if you can empathize with them a little about the cost of food, you may find that at the end of the consultation they suddenly volunteer to make one change, and this will be a very good start.

Summary

A healthy diet is expensive for families on a low income and many feel that it is unaffordable. While recognizing this, those working in the community should continue to educate families about the importance of a healthy diet and in particular about the protective effect of fruit and vegetables. More hands-on experience where men and women are given opportunities to learn cooking skills would benefit many families and provide an excellent opportunity for education.

The elderly are particularly at risk of having a poor diet and should be given advice which also ensures that they continue to enjoy their food.

Key points – dietary advice to low income families

- Try to have some fresh fruit every day
- Choose a polyunsaturated margarine to use on bread
- Try to have a fresh or frozen vegetable every day
- If you can afford it, choose a wholegrain loaf once or twice a week
- Encourage children to drink milk as an alternative to fizzy drinks
- Always make sure that children have something to eat at breakfast before going to school.

Menus for families on a limited budget who have limited cooking skills

The menus below are designed to help families make general improvements to their diets. Some of the meals may not seem perfect but, on a low income and with limited cooking skills, perfection is unlikely! The emphasis therefore is on including some fresh or frozen fruit and vegetables each day and using a polyunsaturated margarine where it is appropriate.

Day 1

Breakfast
Cornflakes and semi-skimmed milk
Toast with polyunsaturated margarine and low sugar jam
Lunch
Baked beans on brown or multigrain white bread
An apple
Evening meal
Cheese omelette, frozen or tinned sweetcorn, carrots and jacket potato
Sugar-free Angel Delight

Day 2

Breakfast
Porridge made with milk
Toast with polyunsaturated margarine and Marmite

Lunch
Edam Cheese and tomato sandwich
Banana and digestive biscuit
Evening meal
Grilled white fish (brushed with vegetable oil)
Parsley sauce made with a packet mix
Mashed potato
Peas
Tinned fruit and custard made with semi-skimmed milk

Day 3

Breakfast
Cornflakes
Toast with polyunsaturated margarine and marmalade
Lunch
Tuna fish sandwich
Orange and a packet of peanuts
Evening meal
Gammon steak grilled or baked
Oven chips
Cabbage and baked beans
Baked apple and evaporated milk or natural yoghurt

Day 4

Breakfast
Porridge made with milk
Boiled egg and a slice of toast
Lunch
Marmite and tomato sandwich
Wholewheat teacake
Evening meal
Chilli con carne (using 2–3 oz mince per person and a large can of kidney beans)
Brown rice
Fresh fruit

Day 5

Breakfast
Rice Krispies
Toast with polyunsaturated margarine and low sugar jam
Lunch
Sardines or tinned mackerel on toast
Orange and a banana
Evening meal
Cheese and potato pie
Cabbage and carrots
Sugar-free jelly and tinned fruit

Day 6

Breakfast
Porridge
Toast with polyunsaturated margarine and marmalade
Lunch
Scrambled egg on toast
Banana and a glass of milk
Evening meal
Fish fingers
Mashed potato
Peas and cauliflower
Blancmange

Day 7 (Sunday)

Breakfast
Rice Krispies
Toast with polyunsaturated margarine and Marmite
Lunch
Roast chicken
Roast potatoes in sunflower oil
Carrots
Sweetcorn and cabbage
Pudding of any sort
Evening meal
Baked beans on toast
A piece of cake

References

Department of Health (1994) *Targeting Practice: The Contribution of State Registered Dietitians; the Health of the Nation*. London: Department of Health

Gibney, M. J. and Lee, P. (1991) Formulation of practical advice for reducing dietary fat intakes in unemployed in Dublin. *Journal of Human Nutrition and Dietetics*, **4**, 179–184

Gibney, M. J. and Lee, P. (1993) Patterns of food and nutrient intake in a suburb of Dublin with chronically high unemployment. *Journal of Human Nutrition and Dietetics*, **6**, 13–22

Mooney, C. (1990) Cost and availability of healthy food choices in a London health district. *Journal of Human Nutrition and Dietetics*, **3**, 111–120

Ministry of Agriculture, Fisheries and Food (1992) *Household Food Consumption and Expenditure 1991*. London: HMSO

NCH Action for Children (Inhouse study) (1991) *Poverty and Nutrition Survey*. ISDN 0900 984

Townsend, P., Davidson, N. and Whitehead, M. (1992) *Inequalities in Health – Black Report and the Health Divide*. Harmondsworth: Penguin

Chapter 12

The nutritional needs of ethnic minority groups

Introduction

Britain is a society which is made up of many cultures including European, Indian, Asian, African and West Indian communities. Since the 1991 census, ethnic origin, rather than country of origin has been recorded so that children from ethnic families who are born in this country are also accounted for. Today approximately 6% of the population in the UK is classed as having an ethnic background and the largest group is from the Indian subcontinent. This is followed by Afro-Caribbeans and then people from Pakistan (Balarajan and Raleigh, 1992).

Geographically, most ethnic communities have set up their homes in the larger cities and in Inner London 26% of the population now comes from an ethnic background. Inner London is home to almost 60% of the Caribbean community, 80% of Africans and many people from Bangladesh. In contrast, Outer London has about a third of the Indian community living there, with others living further north, in towns such as Leicester and Birmingham. Most Pakistani communities live in the West Midlands and West Yorkshire.

Many ethnic minority groups have unfortunately experienced poorer health and higher rates of mortality than their Caucasian counterparts in Britain for many different reasons. Many of them have experienced high levels of unemployment since they arrived in Britain and this, together with difficulties in comprehending a new language, has made them vulnerable to poverty. In addition to this, many people from ethnic minority groups appear to be genetically more susceptible to western diseases, compared to their European counterparts (Balarajan, 1991) and this is also thought to account for some of their increased mortality and morbidity.

Ethnic minority groups are aware that their health is not as good as it should be and this was highlighted in a survey carried out on the health and lifestyles of about 3500 Black and minority ethnic (BME) groups in 1992–1993. In it, the survey found that while only 8% of the general population have described their health as 'poor', 27% of Bangladeshis, 20% of Pakistanis, 17% of Indians and 14% of Afro-Caribbeans described their health as poor (Mori, 1994).

In order to help this group improve their general level of health we need to know more about their lifestyle, and more about their cultural and dietary preferences. This chapter looks at the dietary intake of the main ethnic groups: Hindus, Sikhs, Muslims and Afro-Caribbeans, and highlights the main nutritional problems that someone working in general practice is likely to come across when working with these groups. The following section then discusses the high incidence of cardiovascular disease and glucose intolerance among ethnic groups and the practical dietary advice that can be given to help them.

The dietary practices of ethnic groups

It is difficult to make generalizations about the dietary intakes of ethnic groups as although common patterns can be observed there is often considerable variation between individual families; just as there are among English families. In the section below, dietary customs are described according to the main religious groups but the country or region where a group has originated from is also important in influencing the food people eat. For example, Hindus from the region of Gujarat in India, which is on the coast, are much more likely to eat fish than those from the Punjab.

In addition to this, it must be remembered that all ethnic groups are at various stages of transition into the British way of life. Some, therefore, will have a predominantly western diet, others a very traditional intake of ethnic foods and others still, a diet which is made up of both traditional and western meals. Therefore, while it is useful to keep the general customs in mind an openness to food and culture is also important (Table 12.1).

Hindus and Sikhs

Most Hindus and Sikhs avoid beef, rarely eat pork and only eat small amounts of chicken, lamb, and fish. For many their food intake is based on a predominantly lacto-vegetarian diet and this is generally considered to be very healthy in terms of preventing heart disease. Their main meal usually consists of a vegetable curry sometimes including potatoes, which is usually

Table 12.1 A guide to religious influences on diet

Food	Jewish	Muslim	Hindu	Sikh	Buddhist	Rastafarian	Seventh Day Adventists
Eggs	No blood spots	+	Some	+	Some	Some	Most
Milk/yoghurt	+	Some	Some	+	+	Some	Some
Cheese	Not with rennet	Not with rennet	Not with rennet	Some	+	Some	Some
Pork	X	X	Rarely	Rarely	Some	X	X
Beef	Kosher	Halal	X	X	Some	Some	Some
Lamb	Kosher	Halal	Some	+	Some	Some	Some
Chicken	Kosher	Halal	Some	Some	Some	Some	Some
Fish	With scales, fins and backbone	With scales and fins	With scales and fins	Some	Some	With scales and fins	With scales and fins
Shellfish	X	Some	Some	Some	X	X	X
Animal fats	Kosher	Halal	Some	Some	Some	Some	X
Alcohol	+	X	X	+	X	Not usually wine	X
Cocoa/Coffee/tea	+	+	+	+	+	X	De-caff. are suitable
Other comments	Kosher means food fit to eat by Jewish people, e.g. meat slaughtered in prescribed manner by Kosher butcher. Milk and dairy products not consumed with a meal containing meat. Gap of up to 3 h left between the two	Halal means that the meal contains meat prepared according to Islamic law, i.e. the animal must bleed to death while prayers are said over it	Certain foods are taken during prayers	Some Sikhs may be vegetarian	Some Buddhists may not be vegetarian	Processed, preserved and tinned foods often avoided. Most only eat Ital foods (those in whole and natural state). Fruits of the vine including sultanas, grapes and currents may be avoided	
Fasting	Yom Kippur – Day of Atonement (1 day) No foods or liquids for 25 h	Ramadan (1 month – daylight hours) Fasting involves abstinence from any food or liquids during daylight hours	3 fast days in a year. Devout Hindus may fast on 1–2 days per week				

Reprinted from *Food and Culture* by kind permission from the Community Nutrition Group of the BDA 1995 accompanied by chapattis, paratha or puris made from wheat, maize or millet flour. This is often eaten twice a day and a typical diet is given below:

Breakfast   Cereal with milk or toast and jam
                Tea with boiled milk or carnation milk and often sugar
Lunch   A vegetable curry using onions, carrots, potatoes, auberines, and okra served with chapattis, paratha, puri, bakri or rice
Evening meal Dahl – curry made with lentils or occasionally a fish or meat curry (no beef)
                Chapattis, puri, paratha, bakri or rice
                A glass of milk or some yoghurt, fruit, biscuits, Gur or jaggery (fudge)

Muslims

The diet of the Muslim community depends very much from which country they have originated; however, they are all united in not eating pork and will only eat Halal meat, that is meat which has been slaughtered according to their Islamic rules. This means, therefore, that when they are out they will usually avoid meat unless they know it has been slaughtered correctly. When they are at home, however, their diet consists mainly of chicken or lamb, eggs, and some fish. Meat is usually cooked with a number of spices such as chillis, coriander, garlic and cumin and served with vegetables such as aubergines, okra, peas and carrots or a green salad which may be served with some plain yoghurt. They may eat chapattis, rice, pasta or an unleavened bread called sabayard with their main meal, depending upon whether they are from the Indian subcontinent or north Africa. A typical diet is given below:

Breakfast   Cereal or boiled egg and toast
                Tea or coffee
Lunch   Spiced lamb cooked with tomatoes and aubergines
                Pasta and peas
Evening meal Roast chicken
                Rice and a lettuce and cucumber salad with a plain yoghurt dressing
                Cake

Afro-Caribbeans

Most Afro-Caribbean's have a mixed diet today, which includes both western and traditional West Indian foods. In 1983 the University of Birmingham looked at the pattern of food consumption of Afro-Caribbeans in Birmingham and found that traditional West Indian meals were only eaten every day by 31% of the population (Kemm, Douglas and Sylvester, 1986); today this figure is probably even lower. It is useful, however, to be aware of the sort of foods that they and their families are familiar with, as many of their traditional foods are healthier than the more processed foods that they may have replaced them with from the British diet. In the Birmingham survey, the following foods were identified as being consumed at least three times a week by many families.

- Cornmeal
- Yams
- Sweet potato
- Green bananas
- Rice

Cho-cho a pale green root vegetable and pumpkin were also eaten occasionally, but only by a few families. Afro-Caribbeans usually eat some sort of meat or fish with their main meal and this is very often cooked as a 'one-pot' meal together with rice and vegetables such as peas, cabbage, sweetcorn, okra and plantain.

Afro-Caribbeans may follow one of three religions: Rastafarianism, Christian or Seventh Day Adventists. Those belonging to the Rastafarian group usually try to follow a very natural diet, avoiding processed foods such as tinned products and foods that have had chemicals and additives added to them. Some also avoid pork, fish without fins and scales and fruit that comes from the vine. In the Birmingham survey 47% of Afro-Caribbeans avoided pork, 42% avoided alcohol and 25% avoided tinned foods.

Afro-Caribbean women have had an advantage over women from other ethnic groups in that they have not had to learn English and have had more freedom and independence than many Hindu and Muslim women. This has helped them to integrate more fully into British society and as a result many of them buy a great variety of western foods, compared to other ethnic groups.

Specific nutritional problems experienced more commonly by ethnic communities

Lactose intolerance in adults

In most parts of the world cow's milk is not used in the diet very much and this suits the genetic make up of most non-Caucasian groups who are unable to digest milk. Black and coloured people who move to Europe or the USA, however, frequently find that they are consuming milk and dairy products on a daily basis and for some this can produce unpleasant gastrointestinal symptoms such as abdominal pain and diarrhoea.

Practical advice

Patients from black or coloured ethnic minorities who are suffering from abdominal pain or unexplained loose bowel movements, should be advised to exclude milk and diary products for a month to see if their symptoms improve. Soya milk and soya yoghurts can be used as a substitute to milk and ordinary yoghurt and this will add some flexibility to the diet. If a patient finds that her symptoms have disappeared while following this advice, she should be referred to a dietitian so that her diet can be assessed and a calcium supplement recommended if necessary. If there is no improvement she should see her doctor for further investigations.

Iron deficiency in children

Iron deficiency is widespread among Asian children and is particularly common among the under fives. A few general practices have set up screening and education programmes for Asian children involving a blood test to measure their haemoglobin level and mean cell volume (James *et al.*, 1989). This is taken at the same time as the child attends for part of his or her vaccination programme and if the child's haemoglobin levels is found to be low, the parents are offered an appointment with a dietitian to discuss how they might adapt their diet to include more iron rich foods.

The reason for the high incidence of iron deficiency among Asian toddlers is mainly because of the delayed introduction of solids into the diet. Cow's milk is a poor source of iron and if a toddler is only receiving small amounts of solid food, in addition to his or her milk, they will soon develop anaemia. Some health professionals have recommended that an education programme be set up among Asian communities to promote a more rapid progression through the weaning stages in order to avoid this condition which can delay both mental and physical development (Harbottle and Duggan, 1992).

Practical advice

Parents need to be educated about the importance of iron in the diet; they need to know that without it, a child's mental and physical development is impaired and that iron deficiency can lead to tiredness, irritability and a susceptibility to infections. They should be given written information on which foods are good sources of iron and encouraged to introduce solids at a sensible age. For those wishing to wean their children onto a vegetarian diet, the following foods are suitable and are good sources of iron.

Vegetarian sources of iron

- Eggs
- Pulses, e.g. baked beans, chick peas, lentils and kidney beans
- Whole grain cereals, e.g. Weetabix, brown rice
- Fortified cereals, e.g. cornflakes, Rice Krispies
- Green leafy vegetables
- Savoury manufactured baby foods which show on the label that they have been fortified with iron.

Vitamin B$_{12}$ deficiency in women

Asian women and Rastafarians who follow a strict vegetarian way of life are at risk of developing a vitamin B$_{12}$ deficiency, unless they are very knowledgeable about nutrition and do not have any financial considerations to think of when they are buying food. There have been many reports which have highlighted the high prevalence of megaloblastic anaemia among Asian women, and the deficiency has usually been the result of following a strict lacto-vegetarian diet, together with the practice of boiling milk for several minutes before using it. This practice reduces the vitamin B$_{12}$ content by about 50% and will also destroy whatever folate is present.

Practical advice

Those women following a lacto-vegetarian diet should be advised not to boil their milk and should include some fortified cereals in their diet each day. If this is not possible they should consider taking a vitamin B$_{12}$ supplement.

Vitamin D deficiency and rickets

Asian adults and children are particularly susceptible to developing a vitamin D deficiency and are therefore more vulnerable to the conditions of rickets and osteomalacia. Despite several public health campaigns this still seems to be a significant health problem: in a recent paper in which over 120 Asian patients were screened, over 50% of them had subnormal serum levels of 25(OH) vitamin D and rather disturbingly many of these were women of child-bearing age (Iqbal, Garrick and Howl, 1994).

When people from the Asian continent arrive in this country their blood levels of vitamin D are usually normal but tend to fall during their stay, which suggest that it is something to do with their lifestyle here. Below are the factors which are thought to be contributing towards the problem:

- A reduced exposure to sunlight in Britain
- A poor intake of vitamin D, especially among vegetarians
- A high intake of phytic acid.*

Recent evidence suggests that a lack of sunlight *and* a poor intake of vitamin D are probably responsible for the high incidence of this deficiency among Asians and it is widely thought that the best way forward is to encourage the use of vitamin D supplements. This was certainly demonstrated to be successful in a campaign to reduce the incidence of rickets in Asian children in Glasgow (Dunnigan *et al.*, 1985).

Practical advice
It is difficult for *anyone* to meet the daily requirement for vitamin D by eating the right foods and most of us rely on the sunshine to produce the vitamin D we need. Therefore, while it may be worthwhile spending a few minutes recommending a greater intake of dairy products and fortified cereals to help boost a person's vitamin D intake, it is probably better to spend most of the time advising women to take a vitamin D supplement. This may of course be met with some resistance but should certainly be tried. If women have children, they should be given the following additional advice:

Advice for Asian mothers
1 Give your baby an infant formula milk, at least until they are 1 year old.
2 Give your baby five drops of the DHSS children's vitamin drops every day until they are 5 years old.

General advice for pregnant women from ethnic minorities

Few studies have looked at the diets of pregnant women from ethnic minority groups and so the advice in this book has to be based upon clinical experience and a survey which was published in 1984 (Wharton, Eaton and Wharton, 1984). The main findings of this survey were that the energy intakes of all pregnant women from ethnic minorities were low – below the level set by government recommendations.

---

*Phytic acid, which is present in chapattis, especially those made from wholewheat flour, can bind calcium and vitamin D in the gut and significantly reduce their absorption by the body.

The survey also found that intakes of vitamin D were extremely low in all groups. When individual groups were looked at in more detail, Bangladeshi Muslims, who only ate rice rather than paratha or chapatti, and very few vegetables and fruit, had the lowest intakes of all essential nutrients. So what advice should be given? Nutritional advice can be simplified into three points:

1 Make sure that women are eating *enough* food: check that they are having three meals a day and if possible get them to have an additional snack at some point.

2 If women are following a vegetarian diet, make sure that they are having some pulses every day and 568 ml milk or calcium fortified soya milk every day as well. This will ensure that their intake of protein and calcium is adequate.

3 Make sure that all women from the Indian subcontinent are taking a vitamin D supplement every day (This is now Department of Health policy, Department Health 1991).

Cardiovascular disease among ethnic minority groups

Africans and Afro-Caribbeans

Cardiovascular disease is not as common among Afro-Caribbeans and Africans as it is among those from the Asian continent. However, many suffer with high blood pressure and this is thought to be largely due to their higher body weight (Cruickshank, 1991).

Practical advice
Patients should be encouraged to keep their weight within normal healthy limits and this is probably most easily achieved if they include some of the traditional African or West African foods in their diet. The starchy vegetables that make up their traditional diet such as yams, corn, plantains and sweet potatoes are excellent low fat, high fibre foods to fill up on; and they should be aware that eating some grilled meat or fish with one of these vegetables is much better for them than a beef burger or a piece of battered cod with a portion of chips.

If, however, they prefer a more traditional English diet they should be given advice as to how to make healthy choices.

Asian men and women

Men and women from Southeast Asia are particularly at risk of developing coronary heart disease when they move to a more affluent developed country and it appears that this is associated with their genetic make up (Miller *et al.*, 1988). Although they do not seem to have a greater number of risk factors when compared to Caucasians living in Britain, they do have more risk factors when compared to their own siblings and relatives that remain in Asia. For example, their body weight, serum cholesterol and blood pressure all increase when they move to the UK (Bhatnagar *et al.*, 1995).

Practical dietary advice
Education on diet is important at an early age in this group; men and women should be made aware of the shortfalls of a refined western-style diet and should be encouraged to continue with their traditional foods wherever possible. Their traditional diet of large amounts of rice and chapattis, small amounts of meat and dairy produce and a regular intake of fruit and vegetables, is nutritionally ideal in terms of preventing heart disease; but many Asians now eat a variety of English foods as well and this can result in a diet which is higher in saturated fat and lower in fibre. According to one small study, English foods are most likely to be eaten at midday when processed meats, egg dishes, cheese and biscuits and convenience foods such as pizzas and fish fingers are commonly eaten (Anderson and Lean, 1995).

Dietary advice should therefore focus on the following aspects:

- Explaining to people that many of their traditional meals are very healthy in terms of preventing heart disease.
- Encouraging people to maintain a healthy weight.
- Checking that people are having plenty of fruit and vegetables in their diet.
- Discussing ways in which they could reduce their saturated fat intake, i.e. by changing from butter to margarine and trying skimmed or semi-skimmed milk.

Diabetes in the Asian community

The prevalence of diabetes among English, Welsh, Scottish and Irish groups is over 2%, however among Asians living in the UK it is four times higher than this. This is thought to be primarily due to their genetic insensitivity to insulin, and when they are exposed to a high energy diet they inevitably develop a glucose intolerance. Treatment for this condition is important as glucose intolerance is a significant risk factor for coronary heart disease, especially among women. Patients should be advised to follow a low fat, high fibre diet; lose weight, if that is required, and take plenty of exercise.

Practical dietary advice

Patients should be given the following advice:

- Try to use less oil and ghee in cooking.
- Avoid eating too many fried foods such as samosas, puris and fried rice.
- Keep sweets such as Gur or jaggery for special occasions.
- Continue to use pulses in curries.
- Try brown rice occasionally.
- Cut down on sugar added to drinks.

Summary

Moving from one culture to another has been difficult for some ethnic groups and has brought with it some nutritional problems. Although these are fairly well known among most health workers, some health issues such as vitamin D deprivation and iron deficiency in the Asian community, still remain unresolved. These problems require a renewed effort by those working in primary care.

Many ethnic groups, especially those who are non–Caucasians, appear to be more vulnerable to ischaemic heart disease and cerebrovascular disease and they should therefore be targeted for dietary advice. Ethnic groups should be aware of the risks of consuming a highly refined, high fat diet and the value to their health of a more traditional diet should be explained.

Key points

- Weaning is often delayed by ethnic groups and this can lead to an iron deficiency
- Vitamin D deficiency is common in Asian adults and a supplement should be taken by all Asian women who are pregnant
- All pregnant women should have their diets assessed to ensure that they are adequate
- Education about preventing ischaemic heart disease should be made available at an earlier age
- Diabetes is much more common in people from Asia and India.

Case study – iron deficiency in a toddler

Situation: Jashri Anand was referred with her 2-year-old little boy, Raman, for dietary advice by her health visitor. He had been brought to her attention when he began to suffer from repeated colds and she suggested that Jashri should arrange for him to have a blood sample taken. The result came back showing that his haemoglobin level was only 1.24 mmol/l (8 g/dl).

Diet: Jashri had only recently finished weaning Raman onto a solid diet and this was mainly vegetarian with some fish two or three times a week. He had a poor appetite except for yoghurt and bananas which he loved.

Advice: Jashri was given a list of vegetarian foods rich in iron including peas, lentils, chick peas, baked beans, peanut butter and dried apricots. She was strongly advised to give him a little fruit juice with meals to help the absorption of the iron and to find a breakfast cereal fortified with vitamins and minerals to give him in the morning.

The importance of vitamin D was also discussed with Jashri and she was advised to get some children's vitamin drops from her health visitor for Raman and to continue them until his fifth birthday.

References

Anderson, A. S. and Lean, M. E. J. (1995) Healthy changes? Observations on a decade of dietary change in a sample of Glaswegian South Asian migrant women. *Journal of Human Nutrition and Dietetics*, **8**, 129–136

Balarajan, R. (1991) Ethnic differences in mortality from ischaemic heart disease and cerebrovascular disease in England and Wales. *British Medical Journal*, **302**, 560–564

Balarajan, R. and Raleigh, V. S. (1992) The ethnic populations of England and Wales: the 1991 Census. *Health Trends*, **24**, 113–116

Bhatnagar, D., Anand, I. S., Durrington, P. N. *et al.* (1995) Coronary risk factors in people from the Indian subcontinent living in West London and their siblings in India. *Lancet*, i, 405–409

Cruickshank, J. K. (1991) Cardiovascular disease in black and Indian origin populations. In: *Ethnic Factors in Health and Disease*, edited by J. K. Cruickshank and D. G. Beevers, Oxford: Wright

DOH Report on Health and Social Subjects 41 (1991) *Dietary Reference Values for Food, Energy and Nutrients for the UK*. London: HMSO

Dunnigan, M. G., Glekin, B. M., Henderson, J. B. *et al.* (1985) Prevention of rickets in Asian children: assessment of the Glasgow campaign. *British Medical Journal*, **291**, 239–242

Harbottle, L. and Duggan, M. (1992) Comparative study of the dietary characteristics of Asian toddlers with iron deficiency in Sheffield. *Journal of Human Nutrition and Dietetics*, **5**, 351–361

Iqbal, S. J., Garrick, D. P. and Howl, A. (1994) Evidence of continuing 'deprivational' vitamin D deficiency in Asians in the UK. *Journal of Human Nutrition and Dietetics*, **7**, 47–52

James, J., Lawson, P., Male, P. *et al.* (1989) Preventing iron deficiency in preschool children by implementing an educational and screening programme in an inner city practice. *British Medical Journal*, **299**, 838

Kemm, J., Douglas, J. and Sylvester, V. (1986) A survey of infant feeding practices by Afro-Caribbean mothers in Birmingham. *Proceedings of the Nutrition Society*, **45**, 87a

Miller, G. K., Kotecha, S., Wilkinson, W. H. *et al.* (1988) Dietary and other characteristics relevant for coronary heart disease in men of Indian, West Indian and European descent in London. *Atherosclerosis*, **70**, 63–72

Mori (1994) *Black and Minority Ethnic Groups in England. Health and Life style.* London: Health Education Authority

Wharton, P. A., Eaton, P. M. and Wharton, B. A. (1984) Subethnic variation in the diets of Moslem, Sikh and Hindu pregnant women at Sorrento Maternity Hospital, Birmingham. *British Journal of Nutrition*, **52**, 469–476

Further reading

Community Nutrition Group of the British Dietetic Association (BDA) (1995) *Food and Culture.* London: British Dietetic Association

Fuller, J. H. S. and Toon, P. D. (1988) *Medical Practice in a Multicultural Society.* Oxford: Heinemann Professional Publishing

Polenak, A. P. (1989) *Racial and Ethnic Differences in Disease.* Oxford: Oxford University Press Inc.

Chapter 13

Helping patients to change their behaviour

Introduction

Health professionals are frequently called upon to advise patients on how to change their lifestyle. This may be to help a patient feel better in the short term or with the idea of helping a patient prevent certain chronic illnesses in the future. However, few nurses or other health professionals working in primary care have ever had any training on the subject and know little about the psychology that goes hand in hand with promoting behavioural change.

Behavioural change is a gradual process for most people and there are very few patients who, on their first referral are actually ready to put the advice into practice. For most patients it is something that must be thought about gradually sometimes with over several months and many visits to the surgery.

In this chapter the process of behavioural change is described, followed by a look at how other needs and the need for personal space in a person's life, can make the process of change difficult for people. At the end of the chapter is a section describing how health professionals can make themselves more approachable.

Not all patients are ready to change their behaviour

According to Rollnick, Kinnersley and Stott (1993) the most influential concept to emerge in recent years is something called 'the readiness to change' model. This is apparently based on the 'stages of change' model described by Prochaska and Diclemente (1986). This concept puts forward the idea that people are usually at one of three stages when changing an aspect of their behaviour.

These stages are:

Stage 1　patients who are not ready to change
Stage 2　patients who are considering change
Stage 3　patients who are ready to change.

Patients of stage 1

Patients have different needs at each stage of behaviour change and, if they are to progress positively from one stage to the next, psychologists believe that counselling techniques need to be tailored specifically for each stage (Rollnick, Kinnersley and Stott, 1993). For example, a patient who is at stage 1, should not be overburdened with advice as this could be very off-putting. They will probably welcome some literature to take away with them on the subject but are not ready to discuss the changes in any great detail. This appointment is therefore likely to be fairly short.

Patients at stage 2

If a patient is at stage 2 he is more likely to want to discuss the changes and the implications that these will have on his daily life. Patients at this stage can usually see the benefits of changing but are also aware of the difficulties and they will require more consultation time than those patients at stage 1. Psychologists advocate that these patients are handled sensitively as too much confrontation at this stage may result in a poor outcome in the long term. Patients who are contemplating change often resent being pushed too strongly by health professionals, and it has been suggested that the best way of helping a patient to move forward is to get them personally to articulate the benefits involved in changing (Rollnick, Kinnersley and Stott, 1993). For example, a patient who is being asked to include more fruit in her diet may come back with the retort, 'I should like to, but I can't afford to buy more fruit'. In this situation it is easy for the patient to feel that her circumstances are not fully understood and she may use this rather negative situation as an excuse for not changing.

Encouraging patients to identify the advantages as they see them, is now recognized to be a more successful and less confrontational strategy. For example, in discussing the subject of obesity with a patient, it is likely to be more successful for the patient herself to talk about the benefits of weight loss, rather than the nurse or dietitian. This helps the patient to feel more involved in the consultation and the outcome is likely to be better.

Patients at stage 3

Patients who are at stage 3 are ready to change their lifestyles and are actively seeking information on how to do this. These patients will usually have quite a few questions to ask and will be receptive to advice that is given. At this stage they are ready to overcome any obstacles that may be making the change difficult and will look to you for advice about this.

Movement between the stages

Studies which have evaluated advice given to heavy drinkers and smokers suggest that patients generally move in an orderly way from one stage to the next (Prochaska and Diclemente, 1992). Some may spend several years at each stage, however, before finally reaching stage 3. Patients also have a tendency to move backwards and forwards between each stage: for example, a woman may decide to give up eating chocolate to help her weight loss but may decide soon afterwards that this is too difficult and go back to eating chocolate. Experience shows that she is likely to continue eating chocolate until her weight becomes unbearable again. This see-saw behaviour is very common among patients with dietary problems and they should be listened to sympathetically as no-one likes having to give up a food which they enjoy. It should also be remembered that patients are less likely to relapse if they set themselves realistic goals. For example, trying to restrict chocolate to weekends only, rather than cutting it out all together may be more successful. Again, it is best if the patient can decide how they should restrict their intake, with guidance from the health professional.

Recognizing a patient's personal and social needs

Before discussing the importance of healthy eating with anyone, their basic personal needs should be met. Most health professionals now recognize that basic personal needs have to be met before people can start to think of self-improvement on a higher level and this can apply to many patients seen in general practice .

The concept of ranking a person's needs was first described by Abraham Maslow in 1970, who devised the 'Hierarchy of Need' in which he described three needs: personal, social and intellectual (Figure 13.1).

A person's personal needs include a supply of water, food, oxygen, shelter, rest, activity and some protection from threatening situations or illnesses. When these needs are met, social needs then become important and these include the need to gain acceptance from friends and family members and the

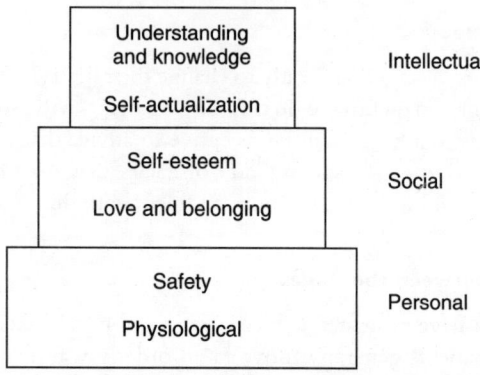

Figure 13.1 Maslow's hierarchy of need

need to give and receive love and friendship. People whose personal and social needs have been met and who have attained a degree of self-esteem in their life are usually much more ready to think about changing their behaviour. However, if a person is struggling to fulfil their personal needs and lacks the security that strong friendships and family relationships can bring, they are unlikely to take their diet and lifestyle very seriously as this is essentially a much higher need.

Therefore, when talking to a patient for the first time, it is important to consider her domestic and social circumstances before deciding whether it is appropriate to give her dietary advice. For example, a woman who has recently had an abortion and split up with her partner is unlikely to be ready, or able to concentrate on any dietary advice at this time in her life because of the other priorities which need taking care of first. In contrast, a woman who is happily married with a stimulating job and no major family problems is very likely to be ready and willing to think about her long-term dietary needs. Time spent with women like this is very worthwhile in most cases.

Acknowledging the importance of personal space

A person's personal space is very important: it allows them to be themselves and to have some personal respect. If a person's personal space is taken away they lose a sense of self-esteem and in the end become depressed.

Illness, particularly chronic illness can result in a great loss of personal space and freedom. It can bring about constraints to a person's life that can be very difficult to cope with. For example, patients frequently find that their social lives are disrupted, that they become more dependent on other members of their family and that life becomes constrained because of the need to attend various medical appointments or to keep to a routine with medication.

Treatment for an illness can, unfortunately, also involve restricting a patient's freedom; for instance if a patient has to give up smoking, alcohol or eating their favourite type of food, they will naturally feel that life has become more constrained and may resent this. If, however, health professionals are aware of this they can try to minimize the disruption that a treatment can have on a patient's life. For example, patients can be recommended to make one behavioural change at a time rather than making several all at once.

Similarly, it is important for those giving advice to acknowledge that there will be some patients who cannot change their lifestyle because the loss of freedom entailed would be too intolerable to them. For example, a woman with pre-menstrual syndrome may feel that giving up foods which contain sugar is too great a sacrifice to make and decide at the end of the consultation that she would rather put up with her symptoms than follow the diet. Although this may seem like a disappointing outcome, every patient has the right to choose this option and their decision should always be respected.

Ways to enhance the process of change

Creating an inviting atmosphere in the clinic

Attending a clinic can be quite an ordeal for some patients and they may have many anxieties about their illness or treatment. Here are some of the more common ones:

- Will the nurse or doctor be able to give me a diagnosis?
- What will the treatment entail?
- Will I have to change my lifestyle?
- Will I be able to afford the prescriptions?
- Will I have to undress for an examination?
- Will I understand what the nurse or doctor is saying to me?
- Will I be able to make them understand my concerns?

In contrast there is very little anxiety felt by the health professional who, in most cases, is carrying out a routine consultation and who is the expert in her field. This uneven level of anxiety which can exist between a health professional and her patient is felt by clinical psychologists to make the development of a relationship more difficult at first. To overcome this all attempts should be made to put the patient at ease, for example kind facial expressions and good eye contact can reassure a patient immediately that you are committed to helping them.

Understanding a patient's expectations when she attends the surgery

A patient's expectations are often different to those of the doctor, nurse or health professional when she comes to the surgery and this can make for an unsatisfactory consultation where each side may be striving to achieve something different. To give an example, a patient with ischaemic heart disease may see her main goal as being referred to a cardiologist, while the GP may feel that a more pressing priority is to persuade the patient to give up smoking. This mismatch of expectations can easily happen when giving dietary advice and it is important to find out if possible, at the start, exactly the sort of dietary advice the patient would most appreciate. This approach is usually more productive in the long term and should encourage patients to come back more frequently for advice.

Similarly, it is also worthwhile checking whether the patient is expecting to see another member of the primary care team and to help organize this if that is what they want.

Summary

As health professionals we need to recognize whether or not patients are ready to change their behaviour. If they are not ready, we must accept their decision and not feel pressurized into persuading them to rethink it. In this way they are much more likely to return to the surgery later for advice. If, however, they are at the point of wanting to change, we must give them plenty of support and wherever possible encourage patients to be involved in setting their own targets as this will usually lead to greater compliance and success.

Key points – helping a patient to change her diet

1 Try to create a friendly non-judgemental atmosphere in the consulting room

2 Check that other domestic and social needs are being met

3 Allow patients to decide, with guidance, which changes they feel will be most suited to their own lifestyle

4 Respect a person's decision to decide at the end of a consultation that she cannot or does not want to change.

References

Eysenck, M. (1996) *Simply Psychology*, pp. 322–324. Hove: Psychology Press

Prochaska, J. and Diclemente, C. (1986) Toward a comprehensive model of change. In: *Treating Addictive Behaviours: Process of Change*, edited by W. R. Miller and N. Heather. New York: Plenum

Prochaska, J. and Diclemente, C. (1992) Criticisms and concerns of the trans theoretical model in the light of recent research. *British Journal of Addiction*, **87**, 825–826

Rollnick, S., Kinnersley, P. and Stott, N. (1993) Methods of helping patients with behaviour change. *British Medical Journal*, **307**, 188–190

Further reading

Jarman, B. (ed.) (1988) *Primary Care*. Oxford: Heinemann Medical Student Reviews

Seedhouse, D. and Cribb, A. (1989) *Changing Ideas in Healthcare*. Chichester: John Wiley and Sons Ltd

Appendix
Suggested diets

Diet one

Description: basic weight-reducing diet: high in fibre, and low in sugar

The first diet is one which is high in fibre and avoids all foods containing significant amounts of sugar. The fat intake of the diet is moderately restricted and patients are recommended to avoid fried foods, pastries, biscuits and hard cheese. However, there is no need for patients to switch to low fat milks or a low fat spread unless they wish to and small amounts of ordinary salad dressing are allowed.

The energy content of the diet works out at about 1200 kcal per day. Calorie counting is not necessary if patients stick to the quantities of bread, potatoes and cereal recommended at each meal. The diet allows a wide variety of foods to be eaten including all types of meat, fish, fruit and vegetables and this should enable patients to follow it for many months without getting too bored.

The diet does not allow for any sweet treats, except in the form of fruit. However, after following the diet for 2–3 months patients should find that they are gradually developing a preference for healthier, less-refined food choices and that they are losing their desire for sweet foods. Some patients report that foods such as cakes and biscuits become very sickly to the palate after this time and this change is important as it encourages a permanent change towards healthier food preferences. This change in the way patients perceive foods is essential if they are to maintain their target weight in the long term.

Patients can expect to lose approximately 1 kg (2 lb) a week depending on their height and weight at the beginning of the diet. This will be more for men and women who are large framed who could expect to lose up to 2 kg a week, initially.

Menu plan

Breakfast
50 g of a wholewheat or oat-based cereal with milk from allowance or 2 Weetabix with milk from allowance
Mid-morning
Fruit from allowance
Lunch
2 large slices of granary or wholemeal bread
1 egg or 75 g cottage cheese or 50 g cold meat or 75 g tinned fish or peanut butter
Salad foods
Fruit from allowance
Evening meal
100 g cooked meat or 150 g fish or 100 g cooked pulses
2 or 3 fresh or frozen vegetables
150 g potatoes or 100 g of cooked brown rice or 100 g of cooked wholewheat pasta
Fruit from allowance or sugar-free yoghurt.

Foods to avoid: all foods containing large amounts of sugar, for example cakes, biscuits, chocolate, fizzy drinks, puddings, etc. Hard cheese, white bread, fried foods, beer and lager should also be avoided if possible and other alcoholic beverages taken in moderation.

Daily food allowances: 284–450 ml ($^1/_2$–$^3/_4$ pint) milk, 3 fruits.

Diet two

Description: a low wheat fibre, reducing diet

There is increasing evidence that there are some people in the population who cannot tolerate cereal products, particularly wheat products, very well (Anderson, Levine and Levitt, 1981; Catassi *et al.*, 1994) and, in my experience these patients do not find the diet above very helpful as it is based on quite a high intake of wheat. These patients on questioning may say that they experienced a lot of wind, loose bowel movements or general abdominal discomfort while on the diet and in most cases their rate of weight loss will be very poor. As a result I have included an alternative diet which can be recommended to men and women who are not successful on the first diet. It still includes a substantial daily intake of fibre from fruit and vegetables including sweetcorn, brown rice and pulses. But does not include any wheat fibre which can cause the bowel symptoms mentioned above. Two slices of white bread are allowed if patients are not happy with ryvita or rice cakes. As with the first diet, it avoids all foods containing significant amounts of sugar and is moderately low in fat.

Menu plan

Breakfast
40 g Rice Krispies or cornflakes and milk from allowance
Milk from allowance
Mid-morning
Fruit from allowance
Lunch
4 ryvitas or 4 rice cakes or 2 slices white bread
1 egg or 75 g cottage cheese or 50 g cold meat or 75 g tinned fish or peanut butter with sprouted beans or salad
Fruit from allowance
Evening meal
100 g cooked meat or 150 g fish or 100 g cooked pulses
2 or 3 fresh or frozen vegetables
150 g potatoes or 100 g of cooked brown rice or 100 g sweetcorn
Fruit or sugar-free yoghurt.

Foods to avoid: brown and wholemeal breads, wholewheat cereals and muesli, pasta, all foods containing sugar, fried foods, hard cheese, beer and lagers. Wine and spirit should be drunk in moderation.

Daily food allowance: 284–450 ml ($^1/_2$–$^3/_4$ pint) milk, 3 fruits.

Note: If patients cannot cut out bread altogether they should keep to 2 slices of white bread a day.

References

Anderson, I. H., Levine, A. and Levitt, M. (1981) Incomplete absorption of the carbohydrate in all-purpose wheat flour. *New England Journal of Medicine*, **304**, 891–892
Catassi, C., Ratsch, I. M., Fabiani, E. *et al.* (1994) Coeliac disease in the year 2000: exploring the iceberg. *Lancet*, i, 200

Index